How to
Be Well
When
You're Not

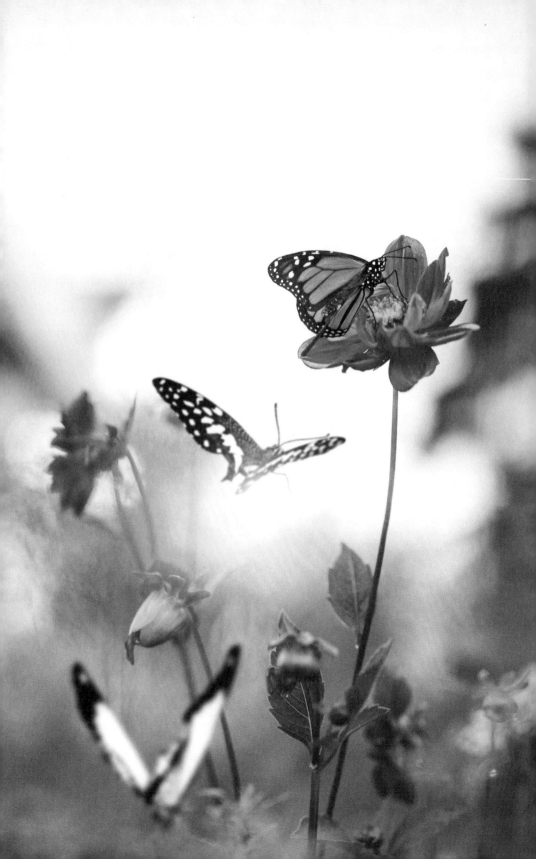

How to
Be Well
When
You're Not

PRACTICES AND RECIPES TO
MAXIMIZE HEALTH IN ILLNESS

Ariane Resnick, CNC

Foreword by P!nk

THE COUNTRYMAN PRESS
A division of W. W. Norton & Company
Independent Publishers Since 1923

DISCLAIMER: This book is intended as a general information resource. It is not a substitute for professional advice. Check with your healthcare professional before you start to include any new food or ingredients as a regular part of your diet, especially if you are pregnant or taking prescription medication, to make sure you are not allergic to it and that it is compatible with any such prescription medication. Do not undertake any new exercise regime unless you are physically fit to do so and have consulted with your healthcare practitioner. Read the Author's Note for additional safety guidelines.

For information about permission to reproduce selections from this book, write to Permissions, The Countryman Press, 500 Fifth Avenue, New York, NY 10110

For information about special discounts for bulk purchases, please contact W. W. Norton Special Sales at specialsales@wwnorton.com or 800-233-4830

Manufacturing by Versa Press
Book design by Endpaper Studio
Production manager: Devon Zahn

The Countryman Press
www.countrymanpress.com

A division of W. W. Norton & Company, Inc.
500 Fifth Avenue, New York, NY 10110
www.wwnorton.com

978-1-68268-346-0 (pbk.)

10 9 8 7 6 5 4 3 2 1

"All of us have special ones who have loved us into being."
—Fred Rogers

This book is dedicated to all my special ones.

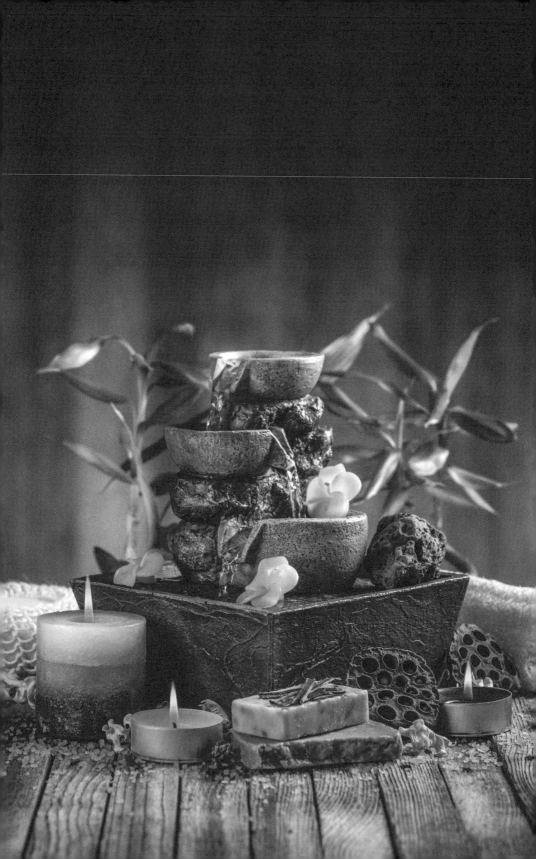

Author's Note

I'm basing the suggestions in this book solely on my own experience with serious illness, and on my consultations with others in the years since. Even so, I do want to put some basic guidelines out there:

- Although Western medicine practitioners turned out to be of very little help to me (and, worse, doctors told me I would never get better), I consulted a large number of them before I turned to other sources of healing, and you should, too. For one thing, you may have better success with them than I did, and for another, they are useful for diagnoses via blood work and other tests.
- Before you embark on any new exercise program, including yoga, check with your healthcare professional to make sure there are no risks for you that you don't know about, and when you do the exercises, make sure you have a thorough understanding of what you are doing. Even stretching can cause injury if it's done incorrectly.
- If you are pregnant, nursing, taking prescription medication, or suffering from any medical condition, please check with your healthcare professional before making dietary changes. Some foods (including herbs and spices) carry serious risks for some people.

- If you use one of the book's suggested ingredients in the form of a supplement powder instead of a whole food, check the ingredients to make sure it doesn't contain anything to which you are allergic and won't interfere with any prescription or over-the-counter medication you may be taking. Also, check for any known side effects! Some supplements can cause very serious reactions, including, in rare cases, paralysis and death.

Contents

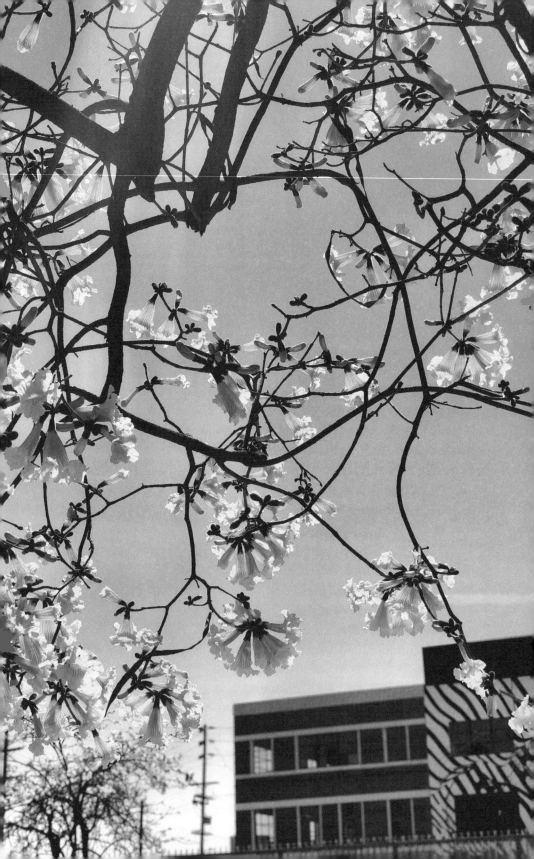

FOREWORD BY P!NK

Food to me is an emotional topic: It is life and I love it. It's an equally emotional topic for Ariane Resnick, the chef and nutritionist who I tasked with feeding me in a way that would get me the body I wanted and needed for my 2018 tour. She was so confident in our first conversation that she could help me achieve my goals, I put myself fully in her hands and we took off on a successful, delicious journey. I didn't think it would be possible for a diet or cleanse to leave me feeling more comforted and satisfied than "normal" food does, but that is Ariane's gift. She has brought comfort to my soul and deliciousness to my life with her cuisine, while also helping me achieve important health goals. Her approach to cooking, nutrition, and wellness is that you should never have to suffer in order to feel better, and that logic has served me in every possible way.

With Ariane's cooking, I never felt restricted, no matter how strong of a plan we were sticking to. She accommodated my array of restrictions, yet every meal was satisfying and nourishing. The first thing I tasted of hers (an Italian wedding soup made with shirataki noodles) immediately became my favorite food. Simple dishes that tasted complex, like her turkey-stuffed peppers and her marinara, made me happy in my heart. Her food had my energy levels soaring even without adequate sleep, and when out of the country and unable to have her cook for me, I followed her nutrition guidelines to keep myself on track as I continued working toward my goals. When I came back, I wasted no time jumping back on her wagon. If I ate just a few of her dishes for the rest of my life, I'd be a very lucky girl.

In addition to her food, which never stopped amazing me throughout our eight months together, the experience of working with Ariane was a joyful one. She made me laugh with her excitement for my meals and the various ways she could make my food world more fun. She even made me cry—in a good way—when she shared how I had positively affected her. It's clear to me that she not only knows her way around a kitchen, but also around getting into a mind-set that will help you be well. She has so much to offer beyond just her yummy food: Ariane is obviously on this planet to help others feel better, and she does it seamlessly. I think it's a perfect fit that she decided to write a book about her journey through illnesses and the tools she uses with clients to help them achieve the same level of wellness that she did. I'm excited not only for the healing recipes in this book, but for how much Ariane sharing her well-earned wisdom will help people's lives. Just as she improved my life, I trust that this book will leave you as a reader feeling better, too.

—P!nk (Alecia Beth Moore)
February 2018

NBD, This Is Just the Book I Was Put on this Planet to Write

What a grandiose statement, right? I initially came up with the concept for this book and titled it in my head when I was sick in 2012. It was the book I was going to write someday, when I was a well person, so that my story could benefit the most people with the least amount of effort on their parts. My thought was that by sharing my experience, I could spare others some of the emotional turmoil I'd experienced in illness.

At the time, I just wanted to feel less alone. I wanted to put something out in the world that other people who weren't feeling well could pick up and read on their couches or in their beds, and that would make them, in turn, feel less alone. Illness is so solitary. No matter how many people surround you, it is difficult to feel deeply understood when you're sick. It's also a struggle to maintain the positive emotions we're told we "should" feel for those around us functioning in perfect health, and that inability can make us feel lonely.

When I got better in 2013, the universe decided pretty quickly that I was going to start consulting others on wellness. Without even looking to move in that direction career-wise, inquiries came in regularly about what I had done and how it could work for others. As I began sharing the tips and techniques that had helped me recover, my desire to put down these modalities in bookform deepened. The more I worked with illness sufferers and the more my suggestions contributed to their wellness, the more I felt this knowledge should be as accessible as possible.

The opportunity to write *How to Be Well When You're Not* didn't manifest until the end of 2017, but I didn't lose faith during those in-between years that it would someday exist. Because this book is the most purposeful, and *by far* the most personal, work of mine, writing it has been a serious undertaking. I gave myself a couple of weeks over the usual six-weeks-or-less time frame that my previous three books took for me to write, but even with a relaxed approach, the process has been an emotional one. In terms of my own path to recovery, outside of the times that are hard to remember, some of the ones that I recall well are painful to recount, and in places my story feels heavy, especially when I consider pitting these stories on people who are dealing with their own troubles.

Never one to be anything but real, which is both a blessing and a curse in life, I'll be honest that this has brought up issues I thought I had grown beyond: Mostly, I've grappled with the worry that I've bitten off more than I can chew in proclaiming that I can help you feel better, because really, who am I? I'm not a doctor or a naturopath. I'm just a girl who has fought diseases successfully and counsels others to do the same. Where I'm normally so confident in life, in writing this, I have struggled with feeling small.

It's taken a lot of continued work on my part to believe, and remember, that what I offer is something unique, that I'm equipped to share it, and that it will benefit you to read about it. Having worked as the chef and nutritionist for P!nk this past year helped me more than anything else to realize that no matter how well known we become, it's totally OK to remain a human-level human . . . and that includes occasional self-doubt. We don't need to think we are the best thing ever to do incredible work; in fact, we stay better people when we are able to be in awe of one another's abilities. Calling to mind her level-headedness, her kindness, her humor, and her respect for me have restored my confidence in this work each time I've lost it. I'm incredibly honored that she wrote the foreword to this, and I returned to it repeatedly as the physical proof I needed that my skill set really is special. Alecia, I have gratitude for you in every cell of my being.

I've done a good amount of pinching myself over what a privilege it is to be sharing my history, my tools, and my knowledge with the public in a more concrete way than the articles, speeches, and podcasts in which I've previously covered some of the concepts contained here. No matter how educated or worldly we think we are, we all must start over repeatedly in our minds with each new undertaking. Imposter syndrome is something that I'm so used to, I don't even bother trying to shrug it off anymore!

So, dear reader, I come to you with this book as a stripped-down, vulnerable human sharing intimate, often unseemly, and sometimes pretty embarrassing details about herself and her past in the hopes that those words, and your ability to relate to them, will aid your wellness. I ask you to be open to new ideas and to be as present as you can bring yourself to be. This journey of mine is now our journey, and I cannot thank you enough for joining it with me.

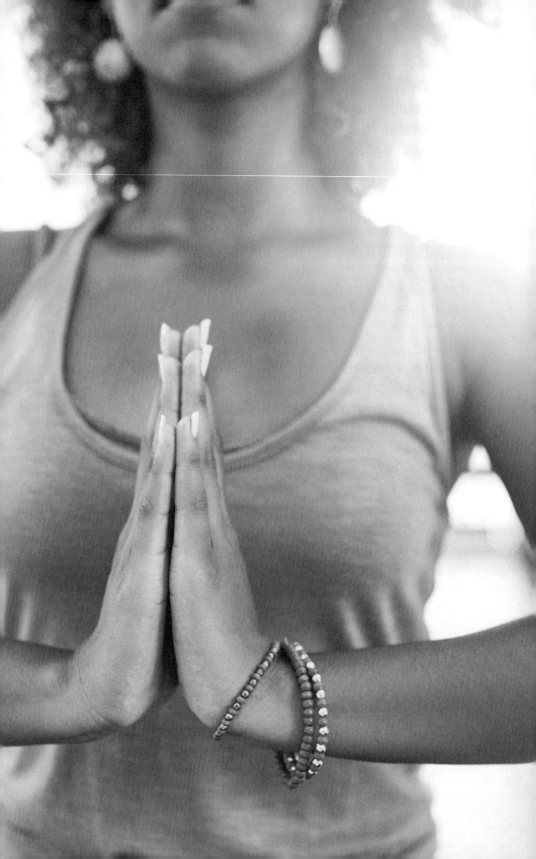

INTRODUCTION
What Is a Wellness Mind-Set?

If you want your body to have the greatest possible capacity to heal, you'll be best served by getting yourself into a wellness mind-set. What exactly does that mean, and how do you do it? A wellness mind-set is the belief, from your aching head to your trembling toes, that you *can* feel better. You achieve it through teaching yourself how to believe that you *can* get well. When you're feeling lousy, it's natural to not have faith in your ability to heal, but it is through that faith that wellness is found. This book is all about getting you into a state where you are facilitating, rather than hindering, your body's recovery capabilities.

When you believe you have the power to recover, you feel less stressed. You experience a sense of hope. You operate from a vantage point that your entire life cannot be summed up by your illness, that there is far more to you. A positive mind-set and the reduction of stress have been scientifically shown to improve chances of recovery.

For example, an article published in the *Canadian Medi-*

cal *Association Journal*, which reviewed 16 studies spanning 30 years, confirmed that patients' expectations of a positive recovery improves the chances of them having one. Dr. Lissa Rankin's *New York Times* best-selling *Mind Over Medicine* is an entire book about how the mind can empower us to heal. There is no shortage of concrete scientific evidence that the belief we can heal helps us to do so. Although this can feel like a new age-y topic, in this book I'll be sticking to the science and real facts so that you begin this next stage of your wellness journey full of credible tools with a scientific basis.

This is a comprehensive wellness guidebook; it will equip you with everything from emotional coping mechanisms, such as how to deal with the changes that feel forced on you from your "previous" life, to mental exercises to help get you in touch with your body in new and valuable ways, to recipes with specific timing, such as a pain-reducing turmeric-ginger tea to sip throughout the day. Through the lens of my own healing, *How to Be Well When You're Not* is my first public, hold-in-your-hand distillation of what I have successfully offered to clients and audiences throughout the world: The relief of knowing that, no matter how you feel currently, you *can* feel better.

My story of chronic illness recovery from late-stage neurological Lyme disease and carbon monoxide/combustion byproduct poisoning is a complex and unusual one, but the challenges I faced and subsequently overcame have resonated with thousands of people around the world over the last several years. No matter how many times I hear, "I'm so sorry you went through that," from others about my sicknesses, I have yet to shed a single drop of the gratitude I hold in my heart for my time spent ill.

Without those health challenges, there is no way I'd be the human I am, with the life purpose I have, of helping others feel better. My illnesses are how I found my calling.

Given that more than 40 percent of the population suffers from at least one chronic disease, this message of mine is one that has no shortage of recipients. I've conducted one-on-one nutrition and wellness consultations via Skype with hundreds of people, have been flown everywhere from Chicago to Paris to help clients learn how to cook for their own wellness, and have trained the private chefs of multiple people (celebrities included) on how to cook in a manner that facilitates their client's health needs without sacrificing taste or presentation.

It was not an easy road for me to get here.

When I made a recovery from Lyme disease that my LLMD (Lyme Literate Medical Doctor) stated was shocking and one of the strongest cases he had ever seen, I thought I'd had my foray with multi-year sickness and would be a healthy person from then on out. Lyme had changed me in ways that felt cosmic, from helping me learn to be a more compassionate person to humbling me about the importance (or lack thereof) of one's physical appearance. However, my feeling like a nicer person did not instill in me a sense of life purpose. And then, less than a year later I fell ill again, this time with carbon monoxide poisoning.

My journey with chemical poisoning made my experience with Lyme look like the flu in comparison. As horrible and debilitating as Lyme had been (I had a spell of fibromyalgia from it that was so bad I required a wheelchair to get through an airport), there were millions of others in society experiencing it too, and there were known cures. Gas leaks are generally fast and furious, and those in buildings with them usually wind up deceased. Being a survivor of low-dose poisoning was something that doctors had no idea what to do with; I was told by neurologists and psychiatrists to "get comfortable," as if I should anticipate a vegetative life.

Seeing Alzheimer's as my official diagnosis on some paperwork when I was 34 years old, and for the first time understanding the gravity of my situation, only increased my determination that my life would not be reduced to my current state. It was late 2012 when that diagnosis came, a full year after the six-month slow poisoning began. Through a combination of supplements that improve cognition and nutrition I made a complete recovery by March 2013.

As soon as I was better, I realized why I was put on the planet: to show others that no matter what they are currently experiencing in relation to their health, whether a minor ailment or a major disease, they have the ability to feel better.

Everything I've accomplished in my career as a chef, nutritionist, culinary instructor, and wellness coach, from working with celebrity clients to writing books to national television appearances, has occurred in these last few years. Once you find your calling, forces align to help you along. I've spoken publicly at length about how our illnesses appear in our lives to teach us the lessons that life tried to teach more subtly, but we didn't learn when presented with those milder, gentler opportunities. I believe our illnesses happen so that we can learn important life lessons. Could those lessons have been learned in a more gentle way? Apparently not, because here we are, sick AF.

When life forces us into ourselves full time, it is what we accomplish emotionally and spiritually that can form a brighter, more purposeful existence after recovery.

I've discussed in interviews an idea I call "the recovery molecule," which is the seed of thought inside ourselves that we *can* get well. I use this as a representation of a wellness mindset because visualization has been scientifically proven to be incredibly helpful for everything from reducing anxiety to enhancing athletic performance. There will be an entire chapter on how to cultivate this concept inside you. I'm hopeful that by parlaying this information, you will not have to go through the pain, bad attitude, and hopelessness that I experienced when sick. If you are already in that sort of state, it should help you make major strides to get out of it!

The food you eat, and your thoughts and feelings about it, also contributes to or detracts from your wellness mind-set.

It's imperative to healing that you feed your body what it wants and needs, not what wellness gurus—myself included!—tell you are healing foods, or what doctors say is best for certain ailments. The food plan in this book includes 35 recipes that work for overall wellness promotion, but my goal for that final section is to get you in tune with yourself so that your diet is one of your many healing tools. When you eat from the perspective of your wellness mind-set, you will gravitate naturally to the foods that best serve you at any given time; you will be less stressed about food (which helps you digest better because you won't be producing the stress hormone cortisol as you eat); and you will feel more relaxed about choosing your meals. Because cooking is rarely something we want to do when feeling unwell, and because illness tends to tap finances quickly, these are simple recipes that don't require strong culinary skills or specialty ingredients.

My guess is that just by reading these few pages, you're at least a tiny little bit excited to learn more about how you can feel better. That little bit of excitement you're feeling? That's your wellness mind-set coming to life. Embrace whatever level of positivity you're feeling right now—it's your key to recovery.

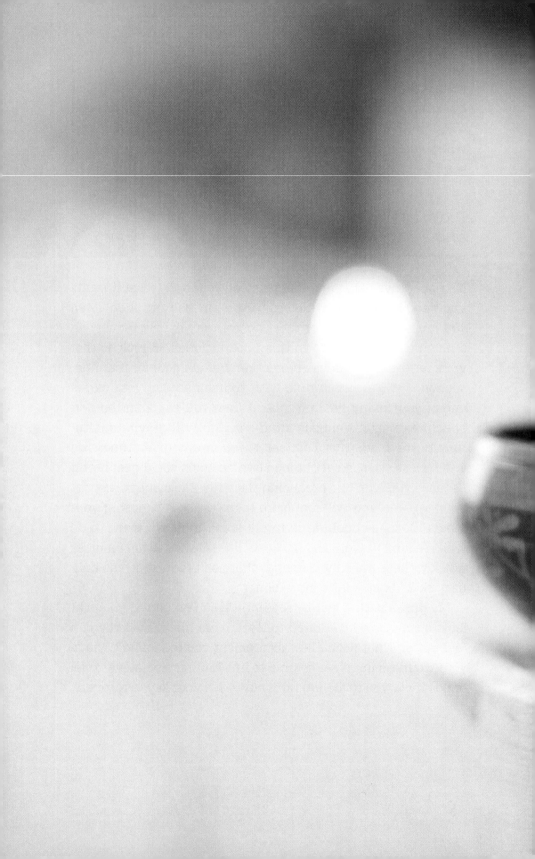

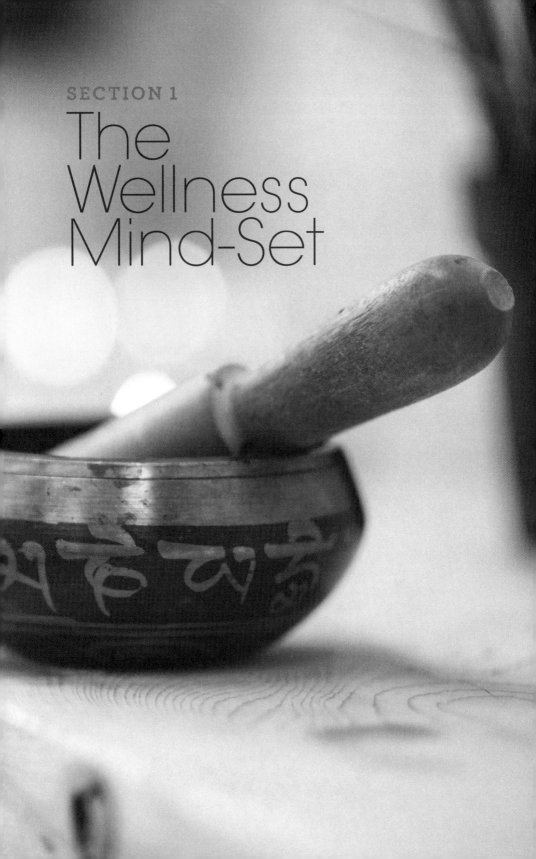

SECTION 1

The
Wellness
Mind-Set

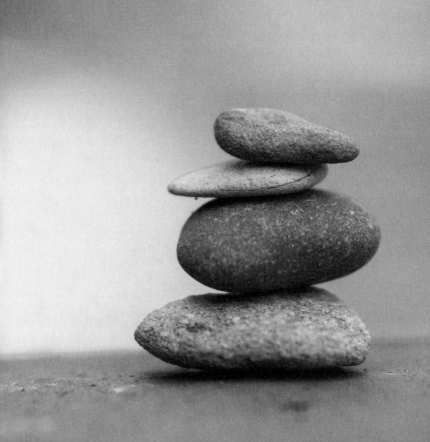

ONE

How My Lyme Life Helped Me Find the Limelight

If you google "Lyme disease chef," my name and/or website will be the bulk of the top results. When I made my recovery from late-stage neurological Lyme, celebrities had barely begun to speak out about it, and when they did, their stories were typically ones of long-term antibiotics and a recovery that stopped well short of them being completely well. "Remission" was the main word used, never "cured."

By speaking publicly about how I not only eradicated neurological Lyme disease completely, but did so without any Western medical treatment, I forged a name for myself in the wellness world far larger than my simple chef and food line background of the time would otherwise have allotted me. I've used the platform of my recovery from Lyme to discuss natural healing, the wellness mind-set and recovery molecule, and much more, feeling that it is my duty to give voice to the potential that illnesses *can* be fully eradicated permanently even if it isn't the norm.

This chapter will go in depth into the emotional, intellectual, and spiritual aspects of my first set of chronic illnesses and how I've used that experience to spread awareness about both Lyme disease and the potential to heal from it—without the prescription drugs that don't even offer substantial cure rates. I will not go in depth about my treatment, nor will I be recommending any specific natural treatments, but will instead focus on how you can use your own illness(es) as a springboard for learning more about your body's ability to heal. My purpose here is not to prescribe supplements or radio frequency machines, but to share my experience of going through an "invisible illness" with a less-than-amazing cure rate so that you can feel more hopeful about your own ailments.

How a Cali Girl Gets an "East Coast" Illness

When I visited Provincetown in Cape Cod, Massachusetts, in the summer of 2008, I'd scarcely even heard of Lyme. I lay in grass and walked around town in shorts and sandals without bug repellant. I did not consider how those small actions would make for a life-changing trip. I did not ever see a little tick on me (deer ticks are incredibly small) or notice a mosquito bite (mosquitoes can carry Lyme too). I didn't get flu-like symptoms, or a bull's-eye rash, or joint pain. I went home from my trip presumably infected—I can't trace anywhere else I was that I was more likely to have caught it, as I haven't been to any areas in Southern California where it's been found—and proceeded on with life as usual for about nine months.

The Downslide

In March 2009, I founded my own line of raw vegan snack foods. The brand, Rawk-n-Roll Cuisine, took off at lightning speed. What started as a small project thought up on a whim quickly overtook my life. To say my product flew off the shelves of the local health food stores they were sold at is an understatement; as new products, they often never even made it to the shelves before being bought up! That month, I worked around the clock to get set up in a commercial kitchen, hire and train staff, and ramp up production to be a viable food business. I had no background as a businessperson, and I did all this setup on my own. My stress levels were through the roof as I waded through everything from legal due diligence and food handler's licensing to packaging rules and regulations.

By April, the dust had begun to settle, and I returned to a more normal level of consciousness in my body. To my shock, I discovered when trying unsuccessfully to zip my jeans one morning that none of my clothes fit. According to the scale, I'd gained about 15 pounds in the last month. My weight had fluctuated in life as it does for many, but at that time I'd been effortlessly about 105 pounds for years, so it was an enormous surprise. Also, that was a pretty monumental gain of more than 10 percent of my body weight, in a very short amount of time. I'd never experienced anything like that before.

As I began to think about other events of the past month, there was more going on than this strange weight gain. I was also noticeably clumsy, which, while never being a bastion of grace, was not a typical problem I had in life. I'd ruined a computer by spilling a glass of water over it, I'd set a tea bag on fire by dropping it onto the stove instead of into the cup, and more. I was feeling even more stressed than I thought I would be, or that made logical sense to be, when starting this business venture, and I was very emotionally sensitive. It was as if I were PMSing nonstop, but the feeling continued to intensify and it wasn't actually related to my cycle.

I'm someone who has traditionally been most comfortable in her body when it is at its smallest, and who has attached a lot of personal value to physical appearance, so the weight gain was my primary initial concern. I began embarking on cleanses

and juice fasts to get it off, but the results were barely tempo-
rary. Juice fasts are known for leading to weight gain after the
loss, but this was happening at super-speed; I'd do a two-week
fast, feel smaller and more energized, then regain the weight
in just a few days. After several of these, they stopped leading
to weight loss at all.

I was stumped by this, and also by my cravings: ever the
health foodie (I was even a raw foodist at the time), all I wanted
was sugar, flour, caffeine, and alcohol. The cravings were of an
intensity I had never experienced, and they were uncontrollable.
Not only would I buy cookies, which was a food I'd generally
only ever make if I wanted them, not purchase commercially,
I'd eat them all and be unable to stop. Multiple times, I cried
as I ate them because I could not bring myself to not reach for
and consume another, and another. Historically someone who
would scoff at a single commercial cookie, I was literally eating
them by the package. My raw foodism was out the window, and
I indulged in junky foods as I never had in life before. The extent
to which I had always maintained self-control over my diet was
one that people had remarked upon for years, so who was this
girl taking over my body? I felt foreign in myself.

Along with my food cravings, my emotional self kept getting further off track and growing problematically erratic. By
summer, I was spending hours on end crying hysterically for
no reason, often in the back of my walk-in closet, while sitting
in a pile of shoes. I couldn't stop crying any more easily than
I could stop eating cookies—I felt the same foreign, overtaken
sense of self (or lack thereof). I also couldn't handle conflict
at all—I went straight from zero to furious, or sad, or, most
distressingly, feeling as if I shouldn't even be alive at all. Not
someone who was ever prone to depression, let alone suicidal
thoughts, this brain in my body was just not my own. I was
managing a kitchen of employees who were steadily growing
tired of my outbursts, which surprised me as well each time

they occurred. I was someone I didn't recognize, and I felt I had little to no control over her. It was terrifying, and I felt helpless.

My physical health was also deteriorating, but not in any tangible way. Beyond the weight I was continuing to gain, I just felt generally unwell. I tried multiple doctors, but was told repeatedly I was depressed, nothing was physically wrong with me. And I was depressed—but only because I felt sick! I had a strong sense that whatever was wrong with me, it was in my blood. I did everything I could think of to purify my blood, such as eating multiple raw habanero peppers a day for weeks. That was miserable, but it didn't have any magical results. Nothing that I tried helped.

The sense of a blood invader was confirmed when I went to acupuncture. Going to acupuncture had hugely improved both a shoulder pain issue and insomnia for me in the past, so I was doing it regularly even though I wasn't able to provide my practitioner with any concrete info about why I was there. At the end of one session, my acupuncturist pulled out a needle from my ankle, and some blood dripped out with it. He was startled, and told me I needed more serious medical attention. "Your blood," he said, "Is orange. And runny." I looked down to my ankle and indeed, what was leaking from me did not resemble normal blood. It was watery, and the color resembled dark salmon rather than cherries. As awful as that was, it confirmed what I knew inside: Something awful had taken over me, and it was throughout my system.

Why Settle for One Diagnosis When You Can Have a Basketful?

I continued trying out doctors until eventually, I struck gold thanks to my ex's research about which illness I might have. In March 2010, I went to a Lyme/thyroid/hormone specialist, and after blood work, I was diagnosed in May 2010 with a host of issues: late-stage neurological Lyme disease, Bartonella (a blood parasite Lyme co-infection), chronic fatigue syndrome (now known as M.E. for myalgic encephalomyelitis), intestinal candida, hormone dysfunction, and Hashimoto's thyroid disease. The doctor prescribed me a year's worth of multiple serious antibiotics to be taken simultaneously, along with assorted other medications.

"Devastated" doesn't begin to describe my emotional state after that appointment. My life appeared to be over, and the doctor, when I expressed shock and dismay at the antibiotics, only told me that after a year of them orally, I might have to move on to intravenous ones. I immediately researched Lyme disease recovery rates only to find out that the intended drugs that would ravage my intestines, joints, and immune system didn't even have a solid cure rate. Lyme was only moderately easy to fix completely when acute, meaning right when you first caught it. That involved two to four weeks of antibiotics, and sometimes people came down with it again later. But when you'd had it systemically for years? The cure rate drastically diminished via Western medicine drugs. Additionally, I had an autoimmune thyroid disease, guts that hated me, and a fatigue condition with no known cure.

My initial response was complete hopelessness. Who could get better from such a long list of maladies? I was overwhelmed, depressed, and saw no way out. Being in my early 30s, it was as if my life had been sucked away from me, and I didn't know how to get it back.

Taking Treatments Step by Step

One by one I began tackling the diagnoses. They seemed less daunting if dealt with individually, stepping back from contemplating the full list of them. Intestinal candida explained my cravings, as it's known for leading to uncontrollable sugar, caffeine, and alcohol consumption. The signals those "bad" bugs are sending to your brain are real, which is why I felt like my body was getting the message to eat such foods in large quantities from some other being entirely. I got the candida under control holistically within a month or two.

I looked into natural Lyme and Bartonella treatment, and started on multiple ones. The only Western medicine I utilized was bioidentical T3 for my thyroid, as I was not confident in being able to cure that naturally, and time-released T3 was a particularly low-harm medication with no major side effects likely.

Unfortunately, the more I looked into Lyme and found other "Lymies," the worse my emotional state became. Here was a worldwide community of chronically ill people who were sick for years on end and were often denied treatment by practitioners. They couldn't work, sometimes they couldn't even get out of bed for months, and they were miserable. It took a good bit of emotional work to understand that those who recover from illnesses don't spend their time on social media discussing them. (That lack of positive voices in the global Lyme community had a strong impact on me, leading me, once I was well, to remain involved so as to be a voice telling others that they too could recover.)

I spent the summer of 2010 using holistic Lyme treatments that left me worse off than I'd begun. Because Lyme inhibits your ability to detox, simply killing the spirochetes (the type of organism that Lyme is) makes you worse, and the detox protocols given for the holistic methods I was employing fell far short of being sufficient. Dead bugs in your body give off ammonia, which makes you sicker.

Within six weeks of herbal treatment, I developed fibromyalgia to the extent that my limbs just would. not. bend. I couldn't even get a glass from the cabinet to pour myself water because I couldn't lift my arms above my shoulders. I wasn't bed bound, but I was homebound. Multiple times I tried leaving my apartment to go to the commercial kitchen and check on my business, which was at that point being run by staff and not reliant on my daily presence. I occasionally made it out the door, but never all the way down the stairs, let alone into my car. In retrospect, it was for the best that I did not drive!

Thankfully, at least my emotional state had stabilized. Going to therapy was imperative for my brain; I'll discuss that more in Chapter Four. Even though I was no longer a raging maniac, though, I was still pretty depressed, especially because I continued only to get worse, not better. When I returned to my doctor for a check-in in September and asked him what my chances were of a full recovery, he said it was more an issue of managing symptoms than ever hoping to get fully well. He said remission was the goal, not a cure, and that it was possible but not necessarily likely to even get to a state of remission. He didn't support my not taking drugs, and felt that my chances of a full recovery were even further diminished by that. We agreed to disagree, and he offered more medications that I did not take.

To manage my pain, he offered me a prescription for Ketamine. A drug I'd only ever heard of as an intense party experience popular in the 1990s (read: K-hole) was now supposed to be my new aspirin. I didn't take the Ketamine, or anything else prescribed. I found a new treatment modality, focused on detoxifying regularly as much as possible, and committed to getting fully well.

I Get Well for a Living

For the remainder of 2010, getting better was my full-time job. I'd moved from hopeless to hopeful through tools like the ones you'll learn about in the following chapters, and there was nothing more vital to my actually getting better than that transition from despair to hope. By the end of the year, I began feeling a little bit alive and mobile. Then, in January 2011, I sprang back to life. Within a month I went from homebound to kickboxing exercise videos. I went back to my kitchen, dropped about 10 of the 15 pounds I'd gained, and felt like a brand-new human. Future blood work would show that while I still had hypothyroidism, it was no longer Hashimoto's/an autoimmune disease, my hormones were able to regain balance, and I no longer had C.F.S./M.E.

When I returned to my doctor in February 2011, he was astounded by my recovery and said it was one of the strongest he had ever seen. Still, when I asked if I could now be considered free of Lyme, he said no; I was in what was considered remission, and would remain that way. Neurological Lyme, he told me, was never considered cured once it has overtaken your system, no matter how well you seemed to be or for how long. He praised how well the modalities I'd used had worked, but said it was still touch and go and to not get too excited about my wellness yet.

Who Knows Best?

I did not let the doctor's skepticism make me any less thrilled to be well or dampen my attitude about the chances of staying that way. I knew I was free of Lyme just like I'd known that I had been seriously sick, long before any doctors would acknowledge it. I continued to do treatment on and off for an additional half year, just in case. Now free of late-stage Lyme disease for at least nine years by the time you're reading this, no way do I consider myself someone in remission; I had Lyme and I eradicated it fully. I'm simply a person who had Lyme, past tense. The disease has the best chance of recurring when you are in an immuno-compromised situation, and less than a year later I would fall ill again in an entirely new way, thanks to moving into a home with a gas issue. The Lyme disease did not return then, and I have no question that I beat it completely.

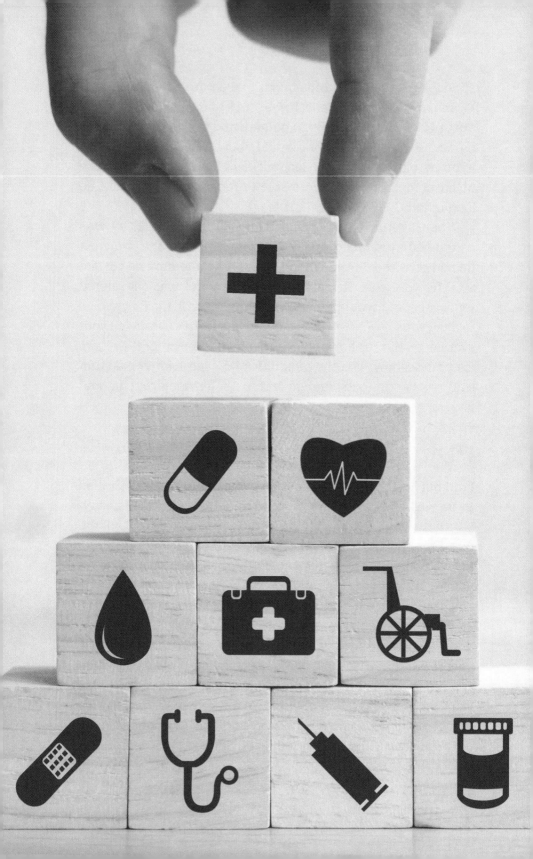

TWO

To Alzheimer's and Back: My Chemical Poisoning Recovery

It tends to be a surprising fact for people that I acquired another chronic illness within a year of getting rid of Lyme disease. Believe me, it surprised the #%&# out of me too! However, I truly feel that it happened for a greater cause. While Lyme disease changed me for the better in a wide variety of ways, which I'll get into when we go over wellness tools in upcoming chapters, I didn't walk away from the illness with any sort of sense of life purpose. I was nicer and humbler than I'd been before, but I didn't feel I had any greater calling. Food was a natural vocation for me, but it didn't feel like I was meant to do it, and I got bored with being in a kitchen every time I landed in one for work for too long a duration. This chapter will detail not only my carbon monoxide poisoning experience, but how getting sick *again* was exactly what I needed to become the person I am now, with the purpose and greater calling I have.

Moving On Up . . . or Down

2011 seemed like it was going to be a banner year: although as a creative person, managing my business financially was beyond my skill set, the customer demand for my brand continued to grow at record speed. I had become the owner of the top-selling brand of kale chips in Whole Foods in the southern Pacific region, and, in total, had gotten my products into nearly 80 stores on both the West and East Coasts. My biggest problem was how much more demand there was for them than I could ever supply, given how labor intensive and costly they were to make, so I began looking into licensing my company out to a larger one. I was glad for its growth, and excited for it to become a bigger success.

I found a company to license my products out to in September 2011 and was unsure what to do with myself once they took over production. I returned to my comfort zone of private chef work out of my home, because I had gained some notoriety as a health food chef thanks to my food line. At the time, I lived in a one-bedroom apartment with my ex and it was fairly cramped between the two of us, so when a three-bedroom unit opened across the hall, we grabbed it.

We had noticed the deterioration of the previous tenants in the past year: three rambunctious college kids who partied loud and hard, they had moved into the unit across from us looking youthful, lively, and beaming. A year later, they were noticeably haggard. When we complained about their noise, which happened multiple times, the female roommate had rage-filled screaming fits at us. We attributed this obvious change in the appearance of each, as well as the craziness of the girl, to their partying. Hey, drugs can take a toll on you! It wasn't shocking that some college kids might have taken things too far. We didn't think anything of it beyond that. They moved out, and into that bigger apartment we went.

What's that Smell?

My ex had a job out of the home, but I was working inside it making food for others, so I was at home most of the time. Within a month or two, she was commenting on a strange fume smell, which we could find no source of, and I was feeling terrible. Her cat, who had had minor kidney issues the year prior but had recovered from them, also took a turn for the worse.

I gained back the weight I'd lost, but it was almost as if I didn't care too much about it; in fact, I uncharacteristically didn't care much about anything at all. I was grouchy nonstop, and my joints hurt terribly. I was constantly hungry, yet food nauseated me and nothing felt right in my stomach. Also, my returned-to-sharp memory started to fail, and my brain on the whole didn't feel like it was working as well as it had been since getting over Lyme at the start of the year. For no reason, I felt anxious much of the time, and volatile. Everyone around me suggested that perhaps I relapsing back into Lyme, but it felt nothing like Lyme had. I knew this was different, but I had no idea what it was.

We began complaining to our landlord that something in our home was making us ill. Mold was the most obvious choice, because the fume smell only happened occasionally and was impossible to track. When we mentioned the odd smell, the landlord suggested it was because we had a window over the building's parking area. Mold seemed more reasonable, and we both knew it as a common environmental issue that made people sick with complex, and often, unexplainable symptoms, so we jumped on that possibility.

Within days, chunks of our walls were being opened and tested. Windows were removed and wooden beams were exposed to find out if the culprit of our not feeling well was living inside the structure of our new home. While one test did result in a positive reading, it was a low enough level that remediation wasn't necessary. Plus, all other tests said that we were within the safe zone, so that test was presumed to have been flawed by a factor such as rain outside.

A Death in the Family

By late winter, I was no longer day-to-day functional. This is a hard period for me to detail because I remember it so poorly, but I know that I wasn't working and I didn't accomplish anything I set out to do, even minor and simple home tasks. I'd try to empty the dishwasher, and suddenly it would be hours later and I'd wander into the kitchen to see all the cabinets open with dishes everywhere. I'd try to get us groceries, but if they were out of an item my ex wanted, I would panic and go home, leaving everything in the shopping cart, often with no memory of parts of the trip. Life just was not working for me at all. It wasn't working for my ex's cat either, who went into kidney failure and ended up dying despite all possible attempts at the kitty hospital to save him.

Diagnoses . . . Again

Because we continued to complain that something in our home was harmful, the landlord sent out an HVAC person in the spring of 2012, a month or two after the cat's death. The HVAC repairman immediately recognized the smell as combustion byproducts from a stove, and thought that, because of where in our home you could smell them, it was coming from the downstairs neighbors. He confirmed this after a quick check of their stove and went into the building to find the problem. The issue was that their stove, which should have been ventilating through pipes outside, was instead ventilating directly into the floorboards underneath us. Every time they turned it on, which was often because they worked from home, we were

flooded through our floors with all of the combustion byproducts, including carbon monoxide, that should have vented
outside. And while Los Angeles doesn't have the coldest of
winters, the entire time we'd been living there it had been
cold enough to not have windows open, so those toxins were
in the air we breathed constantly. To add insult to injury, their
stove wasn't functioning properly, so the emissions were likely
worse than normal.

The HVAC man fixed the ventilation, and we charged forward now that we knew what the problem had been. I con-
tacted an environmental personal injury lawyer and within a
couple of weeks she said she would take the case if we could
get a carbon monoxide poisoning diagnosis from a doctor.

Off we went to the ER, hoping that even two weeks later
our blood would make what we'd experienced clear. Because
of the half-life of CO, we knew it was unlikely we would still
show as elevated. Blood tests revealed that the level of oxygen
in my blood was critically low. As that was weeks later, that
meant it had been even lower while the gas issue was going
on. We received a formal carbon monoxide poisoning diagnosis
from Cedars Sinai, and I was given a prescription for hyperbaric
oxygen.

The Doctors, All the Doctors

Because we wanted to sue our landlord for having exposed us
to toxic chemicals, I followed the lawyer's advice about seeing medical specialists to prove our case. Unfortunately, none
knew what to do with me. Carbon monoxide generally kills; it's
rare for someone to be exposed to low doses slowly and survive
it. Also, the other combustion byproducts I'd been breathing
nonstop for half a year? They create a range of symptoms too,
but again, this was a field no medical professional knew anything about.

I did a month of daily hyperbaric oxygen, only to end up feeling worse and experiencing, no joke, oxygen toxicity from too much hyperbaric oxygen. I saw a cardiologist to find out if the heart condition I'd had since childhood had been worsened by the CO, and actually had to read to him about how carbon monoxide affects the heart via a Google search I did, because he knew nothing about it. I saw a neurologist for my nonstop migraine, and he suggested migraine medication. When I asked him how I'd know when the migraine would eventually go away while I was on the medication, he had no answer. Doctors were a source of frustration instead of assistance, which felt eerily familiar to my early days of Lyme. How had I landed in this situation *again*, not even two years later?

The neurologist sent me to a psychiatrist for cognitive testing, as it was important to prove my brain deterioration via a professional. The testing took many appointments, totaling more than 10 hours, and showed that I was basically a disaster. Once a girl with a genius IQ, I was not so far above brain dead now, and I had all kinds of kooky personality disorders, too. Anxiety, panic disorder, and depression were just a few of the labels that fit my state. I was devastated, to say the least, not only with the diagnoses but with how little hope there seemed to be for me.

Months later, the neurologist would order a CAT scan of my brain to see if the damage was visible. When I saw "Alzheimer's disease" as the diagnosed illness listed for the reason behind the image request, I was floored. I knew things were bad, but Alzheimer's?!?! I was basically being called senile. At the age of 35, no less! How was this my life?

The CAT scan did not show anything definitive. I asked the neurologist what I should do, and his response was to get comfortable. I was written off by Western medicine as a hopeless case, and I did not see him or the psychiatrist again.

Ms Resnick **DID** have difficulties in the area of non-verbal reasoning. It appears that Ms Resnick scored within the **LOW AVERAGE RANGE** in her ability to understand the meaning of visual or abstract information and recognizing relationships between visual-abstract concepts.

Summary and Conclusion

Ms Resnick neuropsychological report **DID** reveal some important information. It appears that **Ms Resnick is having some memory difficulties** in the areas of visual recognition, proactive interference, complex visual memory skills, higher order cognitive processing, spatial and visual memory, processing of linguistic information and perceiving social information. Ms Resnick also is not using the most effective learning strategies such as semantic clustering but rather seems to be using haphazard methods in remembering words.

Psychologically, Ms. Resnick can be considered to have a Diagnosis of generalized anxiety disorder and obsessive-compulsive disorder which are most typical with her MMPI profile. In addition, a diagnosis reflecting conversion elements would not be ruled out. Diagnoses of depressive disorders are also seen with this pattern along with diagnoses of dissociative disorders. Secondary diagnoses of dependent personality disorders are also common.

Treatment Recommendations:

1) **Memory Treatment Program** – Ms Resnick would greatly benefit from a cognitive intervention to improve her memory and abilities and neuropsychological wellbeing. The program being suggested is the **Memory Treatment Program** by Scientific Brain Training PRO. There are specific exercises to treat memory impairment. Exercises in this program have been utilized by the Alzheimer's Treatment & Memory Training Centers of America for nearly a decade to treat patients suffering from early stage Alzheimer's disease and Cognitive Disorder and other causes of memory impairment.

2) **Neurological Evaluation** – Continued evaluation by Dr. Singh to determine if there is any progression of her cognitive issues.

3) Psychotherapeutic Intervention- Ms Resnick should continue her work in psychotherapy.

My Return

Life continued this way throughout the remainder of 2012. I tried different holistic healing diets and was able to get rid of the physical symptoms of the poisoning, such as my extreme joint pain, as well as my digestive issues. Eventually, and again with my family's help, I found the right combination of food and supplements to heal my trauma-ridden brain. Similar to the same time of year as Lyme disease, only two years later, at the start of 2013 I began my recovery from chemical poisoning.

By March 2013, I was functional and decided I was ready to reactivate a chef profile on an event website that had asked me to join the year prior, but whom I'd never worked through because I was too sick. The day after I made myself available, the website itself called me about a collaboration they were doing with Goop, asking me to cook for Gwyneth Paltrow for the day.

I gave an enthusiastic "Yes!" to the request despite having never successfully cooked meat before (I'd been a veggie chef for the duration of my on-and-off chef career and generally failed at trying to cook it for people I was with). I did well enough on that one-day gig that they asked me to be their chef and I've never looked back since.

Purpose Found

When I was in the process of getting better from chemical poisoning, it was incredibly important to me to figure out why I'd gotten so sick again in the first place. That the point of my illness was for me to find a sense of purpose was something I felt deeply, mostly because it was the only thing that made sense. While Lyme had taught me how to be nicer and less judgmental, it hadn't even occurred to me that holistic healing, and my ability to recover from a major illness with only natural methods, was something special.

I realized through chemical poisoning that we are all here to recover; sure, we are meant to thrive, but no life is led only in good times! We are here to get better and to pick ourselves up from whatever knocks us down, no matter how many times we get knocked down . . . and sometimes, for years at a time even, it feels like all life does is knock us the %*^&# down! My ability to recover felt, on a deep level, like something that I should be sharing with the world. Food and writing are my natural vehicles for expression: I never decided to cook for work, just like I never decided to write for work. They are the activities I perform when no one is paying me to do anything; they are my second nature. That I have a life in which the things I do as hobbies are also what comprise my income is an incredible gift I thank the universe for daily.

Putting two and two together with food and wellness as a career path was, well, about as easy as putting two and two together and coming up with four. As I got better from the chemical poisoning, I realized that I am here to share my ability to get well with others looking to do the same. I'm here to show people that a life well lived doesn't mean an easy life, or a life free of strife or illnesses—it means a life in which no matter what happens, you get up for the next round and you give your all, over and over again.

I began doing chef work with an even more holistic focus than I had in the past, and I opened up to the possibility that my B.A. in Creative Writing might finally be of use. Within two years of my return to working, my first book was offered to me by a publisher. What you are reading is my fourth, and in this time, I've also written countless articles on nutrition, food, and wellness, as well as spoken at a good number of conventions.

I'm 100 percent confident that without my illnesses, I wouldn't have found this path. What I learned by being sick was immeasurable, and I'm not exaggerating when I say that really, I wouldn't take back either experience. They made me who I am, and I like this person a lot better than the one I was before. If you follow the tools contained in this book to help you be well when you're not, I think you will prefer your future self, too.

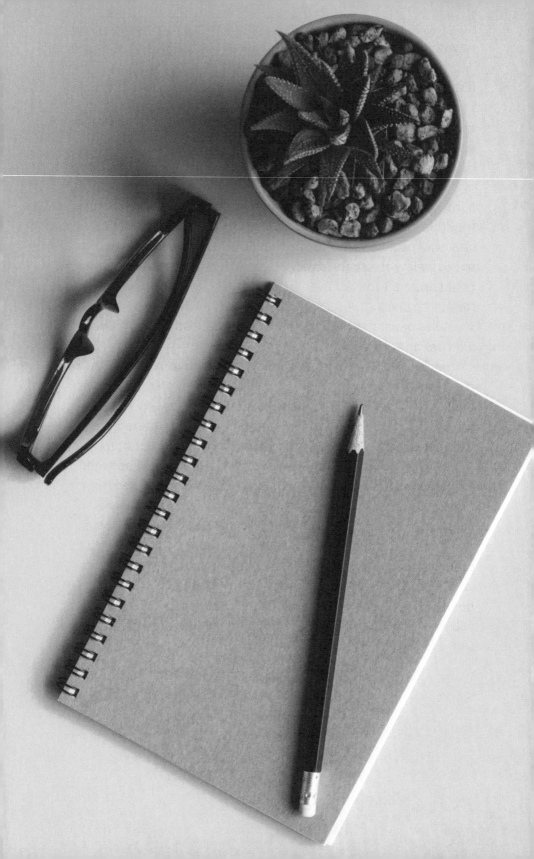

Healing Assets

In this section of the book, you'll be doing an assortment of written exercises. I recommend that you keep a wellness journal so that all your work is done in one place. Any notebook will do! You may wish to leave pages of space between exercises so that you can go back and do different versions of them later, as many have a good deal of choices to pick from. The more you do them, the more you'll be facilitating your recovery, so don't worry about overdoing any.

For all exercises, please read through the directions before beginning.

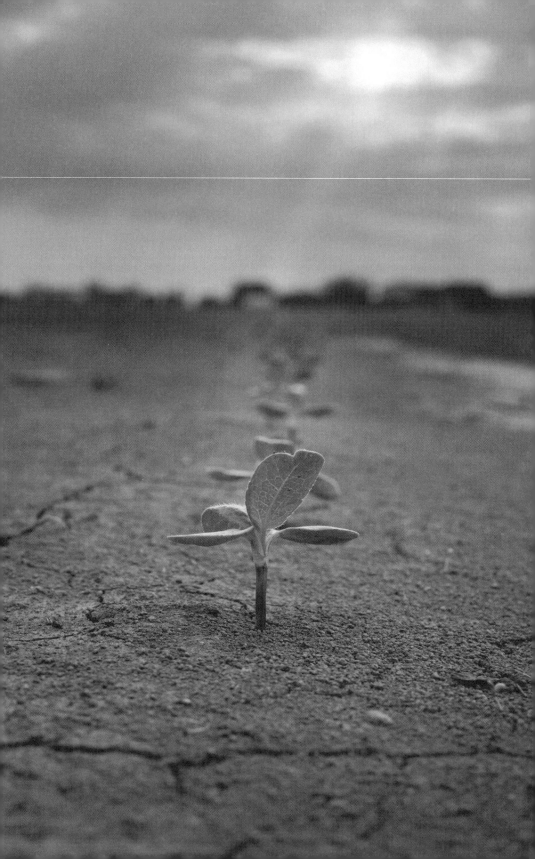

THREE
The Recovery Molecule, and How to Find Yours

The Survival Piece

No matter how easy or difficult your life has been, you've inevitably faced many challenges, and at any point, you could have given up and called it a day on this existence. You're here because something inside you told you to keep on living, and propelled you forward when your conscious mind could not. Survival instinct spans, as far as I can tell, pretty much all life forms. From algae to alligators, while alive we generally will do whatever it takes to keep on living. This instinct works whenever it's needed, regardless of whether we are princes or paupers, from the age of consciousness until too old to hold on any longer, and with very rare exceptions.

Your survival instinct is primal, similar to the quest for food when hungry or the migration to shelter in the rain. We would never have made it this far as a species without it, and whether you credit natural selection or God or the forces of the universe, the will to live is one of the strongest, if not the strongest, instinct we have.

It's not, however, enough on its own—at least not all the time. You can be sick for years, and you're still surviving. But are you really living, in a way you're happy about? Do you feel like your life is worthwhile? Do you have things you look forward to? Are you excited about tomorrow, or the day after that? I hope the answer to all of these questions is "yes," but I understand if it's not. Surviving doesn't mean thriving, and it doesn't mean feeling like life is worth living. It means you haven't given up completely, and while I'm really, really glad you haven't, you probably agree with me that still breathing is not enough. How can you build on this survival instinct to get well? I'm happy to show you that there are many ways to bolster it!

The Love Piece

Entirely different, yet inextricably tied to our will to survive, is our ability to know love. We experience love all throughout our lives, and in countless forms. There is love for our families, given without any conscious thought right from the start of our lives; later, there is love for our friends, significant others, and mentors. There is love for food, entertainment, material possessions, and experiences. What we love is a big part of what makes us unique humans, and there are no two people who love only the exact same things as one another.

We can love all sorts of things, from other people to the taste of chocolate, but we also know love in a deeper way. It is no coincidence that so many stories in our cultural imagination have love as a motif. Whether it is what saves the world or saves a person, and whether it is overtly in the plot or contained in the subtext, love is a major theme in our books, movies, and songs. And you know what almost always happens? It wins. If love hasn't won, the story probably isn't over. That relates to you, too: If you haven't found your depth of love, your story is still being written, too.

On the one hand, no matter how many people we do or don't surround ourselves with, when you go to bed at night it's just you residing in your brain. But on the other hand, we all, whether or not we are in touch with it, have a sense of a deeper connection to one another. "We are one" is a statement spoken through time immemorial, in myriad cultures. There is something inside us that longs for connection to others, and we all have the ability to feel that connection to our greater consciousness, no matter if there are other people physically around us. The love piece of the recovery molecule is the act of being in touch with that feeling of love; it exists tangibly at any given moment.

Survival + Love = The Recovery Molecule

It is awesome to know that these two deeply vital parts of existence can combine to help you believe you can get better—so how do you go about getting yourself to a mental place where you're actually believing it? As with most wellness tools in this book, there is no shortage of ways to find your own belief in recovery!

Ignore 'Em

Funny topic line, huh? Unfortunately, much of what we hear from professionals about our potential for a full recovery is often not very hopeful at all and can leave us figuring we might as well resign ourselves to a lifetime of illness. I literally got told, "Go get comfortable!" What will believing that you may not fully recover do? It will keep you sick. Yet over and over, we buy books and watch stories of people who have overcome the odds, because we know it's possible. What's preventing you from thinking that you, too, can overcome them? All of those other people whom you might think are better, or stronger, or smarter, are truly no different than you are. They are just people who found their versions of the recovery molecule.

With both of my illnesses, I had things said to me about how slim my chances were of ever being completely well again. On each new occasion they were uttered, I started to believe those sentiments more and more . . . and boy, was that freaking horrific. Granted, your life will never be what it was before, but that's because time moves forward, and whether you're sick or well, it will never exist as it did in the past. (We'll get into that more in Chapter Five: Finding the Lessons in Illness.) Even if you have had a major situation such as a body part amputated, there are survivor tales of others who had experienced something similar and went on to lead happy, fulfilling lives.

The easiest and first tool to believing you can get well is, therefore, very straightforward: ignore those who tell you it isn't possible. The world is full of people, myself included, who got better after being told they wouldn't. I had an Alzheimer's diagnosis, yet here I am typing out tens of thousands of words to you; I had fibromyalgia so bad I couldn't walk through an airport, but this morning I did an intense H.I.I.T. workout followed by a spin class; I couldn't digest anything beyond rice pasta and salad greens for months, and here I am having just devoured a delicious peanut butter protein cookie I made. "Anything is possible" includes you! You are not exempt from this rule, and there is no limit or cap on how many people can get well after being told it's not likely. Health is an unlimited pool.

How do we turn this idea into a quantifiable exercise you can do right now? Just follow these steps to begin changing your mind-set today.

Eraserhead

Close your eyes and picture one of the professionals who has told you that your chances of recovery are anything short of 100 percent. Envision this person clearly and hear their words. Now, take a giant eraser in your mind and white out their body from the background where they were when they told you this. As you erase their mouth, silence their words. You can even mentally speak over them if helpful, saying, "Shut up," or, "I can't hear you," or, "I'm not listening to you."

In that room, there is now space for a person. Put someone there whom you love and trust, and hear them tell you they believe in their heart that you can be well again. If it works, you can put yourself there, as you are the highest authority on yourself that exists.

Who else would tell you that you will make nothing short of a full recovery? Repeat this with as many characters as you need to. Do this as many times as you'd like, reveling in the erasure of something that you don't have to allow to be your truth.

What Matters

It is natural for you to not feel connected to the cosmic sense of togetherness, so here is another helpful exercise that will get you in touch with that love feeling I was talking about.

First, in your wellness journal, make a list of the things that matter the most to you in life. There are no right or wrong answers here. What's most important to you could be solving world hunger or it could be your favorite T-shirt—it doesn't matter. No one is judging you, and really, what is there to judge anyway? Your priorities make you uniquely you, period. Leave several lines of space after each item you choose.

Next, in the empty space after each item, write down how you personally relate to it; this is so you can understand how

you are a part of it, even if you are not experiencing it right now. For example, if the most important thing in your life is your children, they do not need to be in the room with you right now for you to relate to them. They are a part of you through your genes, through the lessons you have taught them, and through the love you have given them. When you think of a memory of them, you can feel their love for you. Even just by calling them to mind without a specific memory, you can probably feel their love for you. I know I can feel my mom without doing anything except bringing up the thought of her.

These feelings are a higher, and deeper, connection that goes beyond just us in our daily lives. The love you feel for your children does not stop when they leave home, or when they misbehave. It is larger than that. The love you have for your children is you being tuned in to a greater sense of love, and it is through your children that you are feeling that cosmic sense of love. They are the conduit for, and a representation of, a love that exists inside of you and it is bigger than any one human, whether they sprang forth from your genes or not.

This works for people, concepts, objects, anything. What you are looking to do here is gain the understanding that what is important to you is, yes, things and people and ideas, but also the way they make you feel connected to love overall.

It might not come naturally to detail how you relate to your priorities, and that's OK. Think on each item for as long as you need, and by the time you have related each to yourself, you should have at least a mild sense of that great big concept of love that goes way beyond any of us.

The Opposite Game

Because you've probably heard a lot of negative things about your health, and because those thoughts are likely stirring endlessly in the ever-expanding pot of your brain, we're going to defuse their power by flipping them on their heads.

Think of at least three sentences you've been told by professionals, be they diagnoses or prognoses, and write down the opposite of them. This looks as simple as, "Mrs. Smith, you do not have Parkinson's disease," or "Mr. Johnson, you will probably live well into old age," or "Susie, your blood work is perfection. You are a pinnacle of health."

When you write down these opposite statements, do your best to hear them in your mind. Maybe even say them aloud to yourself, to know how good they feel to hear. Feel into the experience, really putting yourself in the situation like you were when it happened the first time, only this time, all news is good news. You will be well. You can be well. You are well.

Avoid writing down the initial statements to avoid giving power to them through your written word. An exception here can be made if your brain function is decreased to an extent that unless you write down the original, you can't think of the opposite. If that's the case, go ahead and record both, and once done, draw thick lines through the original negative statements.

Self-Talk to "You"

For your best chance of finding your belief in recovery, you'll need to be speaking to yourself as a person who has the ability to recover. You can't tell yourself something is the truth and a lie at the same time; your internal conversation needs to involve you talking to yourself in a way you can believe. It takes a lot of practice to remove negative self-talk, but being kind with yourself, believing in your value as a person, and in your ability to feel well again, are all necessary parts of actually returning to wellness.

Sometimes it can be difficult to believe what we say to ourselves when we speak in the first person, compared to the second. It can be hard to believe "I am getting healthy," but when we say it to ourselves as "You are getting healthy," as if it were another person saying it to us, we may be more inclined to internalize it.

Take steps to shift your internal self-talk into the second person and see if that lightens the burden of belief for you. I can't tell you how many times I've said in my own mind, "Ariane, you've got this!" in order to find the courage to do something scary or intimidating. It's a tip I picked up from a neuroscientist named Dr. Robert Cooper who spoke at the same Bulletproof Conference as I did a few years ago. I loved his perspective about how you can make your life better by changing the ways you think about things, and I immediately began employing this technique. While I do still think in the first person/"I" as a default, whenever I need to give myself encouragement, I've practiced the second person/"you" enough for it to be how I word that messaging internally. His suggestion of using your name is one I employ often, as it makes it all the more powerful.

Lofty Goals Are the Best Goals

By moving through these exercises, you should be slowly getting in touch with your inner recovery molecule, and moving from a mental place of seeing healing as a remote possibility to a place where it is viable. When you are able to have a sense of belief in your ability to heal, strengthen it further by imagining what you will do once you're better. We'll get more into this concept in Chapter Five: Finding the Lessons in Illness, but this is a good place to introduce it and to plant the seed of planning your post-illness life.

Too often when we think about feeling well again, we imagine ourselves in the past, before our ailments. This is, of course, not how life works, and visualizing the past will not lead to a better future. No matter what, life goes forward; that happens regardless of your health. Spend a few moments thinking through your recovery process. Imagine that little recovery molecule spark inside you, growing until it becomes the guiding light that leads you forward. What begins to change in your life as you feel better? What are you most excited for? Where will you go that you can't right now? What clothes will you wear, what food will you eat, who will you talk to, what physical activities will you take part in? The world is your oyster; feel into that. Breathe into that as many times as you need to until somewhere inside of you, some tiny little piece of you believes it. That tiny little piece of you, that tiny little spark, it is real, and it contains everything you need to be well.

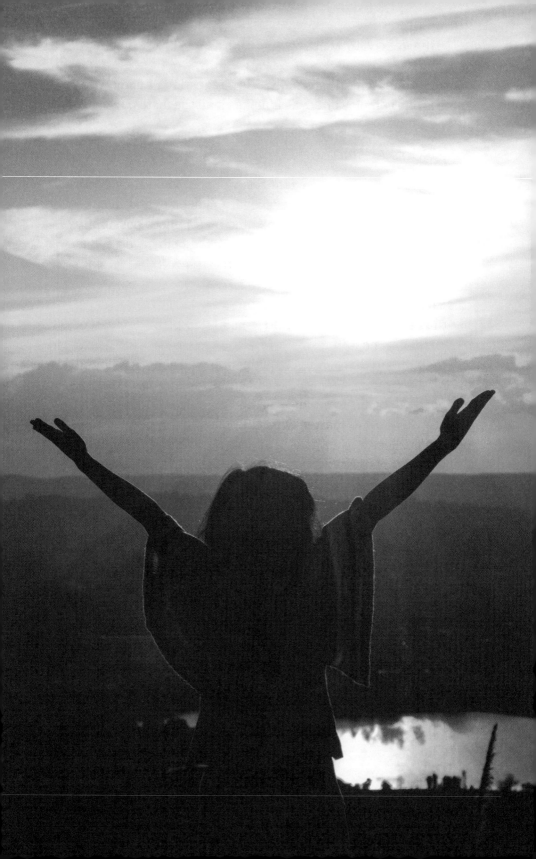

FOUR
Befriending Your Body

We all have moments in our lives where everything suddenly changes. You cannot anticipate these instances, nor can you prepare for them. The most you can do is recognize an epiphany when it happens and run with it to the best of your ability. I attribute much of my Lyme disease recovery to just such an epiphany.

When Doctors Do Know Best

Behavioral therapy played a huge role in my dealing emotionally with Lyme disease—it's normal for neurological Lyme to offset your emotional state, as the spirochete (Lyme organism) can migrate into and live in your brain. While sick I found myself, previously sound emotionally, someone who would curl up in a pile of shoes in the back of her closet and sob hysterically for hours, over absolutely nothing.

I'd often wake up in the middle of the night crying and unable to stop, and I went from being very in control of my emotions and anger to experiencing "Lyme rage," which is the term used in the Lyme community for an uncontrollable anger that comes out of nowhere and is incredibly difficult to control, especially for people with no previous anger problems (and therefore, no tools for managing extreme anger). Despite never having had suicidal thoughts before, the moment my life had any sort of conflict in it, the foremost thought in my brain was that it would be easier to not be alive. I thought I was being rational, and that finding an escape to the solution would be my best bet. Thankfully, those thoughts were only thoughts, and I never did anything physical to take action on them.

Therapy taught me how to separate my symptoms from who I was as a human, and only a short while into learning that process, I was able to regain control over my emotional state. It was in my first session that my therapist helped me separate the two, by reviewing with me behaviors that were mine versus those that were Lyme related. This is a tool that can be very helpful.

You Are Not Your Symptoms

Take a moment to pause from reading and evaluate the behavioral changes in yourself since you got sick. Are you moodier now? Are you sad or depressed? Have you given up hope on life? Do you have bursts of anger? Do you cry more than you used to, or not at all anymore? Do you feel resentful of your friends for their wellness, to the point that it makes you angry? Are you envious of "normal" people?

All of these emotions, and more, can go along with illness. Whatever the ailment, illness can change our biochemistry so much. Serotonin is mostly produced in the gut, and it's rare to have a major health problem yet a strong gut and immune system. It's important now to remember who you are at heart. Which of these questions that you answered "yes" to feel like that's not the person you once knew yourself to be? Passing something off as a symptom of illness isn't passing the buck on responsibility, but rather acknowledging how your circumstances have changed your outlook and behavior.

For any behaviors that aren't "you" deep down, you should recognize the incongruity and be able to feel, at least a little bit, that the version of you expressing yourself is not who you are spiritually. Once you have examined and recognized those behaviors, forgive yourself for them. The realization that they aren't you is the first step needed to changing them!

From here on out, when you find yourself about to act angry, depressive, or anything else that isn't your nature, take a deep breath and realize these thoughts are the illness talking. Look inside instead to find how you really want to express yourself. My guess is that the person you were and want to be is kinder, gentler, and more able to control their temper.

The Miracle Moment

I saw my therapist regularly throughout my illness. One morning in December 2010 I had a phone consultation with her because I was too ill to drive. She asked what was foremost on my mind, and I told her that I felt I was at war with my body, and I could not win. She said to me, "The only way to win that war is to not fight. Befriend your body, and it will befriend you." The notion that there is something in our bodies that we must kill, fight, demolish, and/or ruin creates an internal environment of turmoil and struggle, and that is how we typically frame illness. Being told to step back and find light instead felt like the opposite of my instinct, and I somewhat dismissed her suggestion as a bit too hippie for my taste.

After my session, I got up from my bed to use the bathroom. When I looked in the bathroom mirror, the person staring back at me was someone else: I had a vision of who I would be after Lyme disease. The girl I saw in the mirror was kinder than I had ever been. She had compassion. She was grateful for her body's pain-free existence. She did not judge others who were less book smart. She did not fret over how every food would or wouldn't hurt her stomach. She was free. She was well. She was happy.

It was a flash: I blinked once or twice, and my sick self returned to the mirror. But it set something off inside me that felt like an epiphany. I *was* going to get better, and I was going to do it *now*. The treatments were going to work—hell, they *were* working. I was going to be this person I had seen in the mirror, and I was going to lead a happy, gratitude-filled life.

Recovery: Set in Motion

About a month later, as mentioned in Chapter One, I was back to working at my food business (which had been run by staff without me for countless months) and following along with kickboxing videos. I'd gone from laid up for nearly two years to completely well over the course of about 30 days after that session. The holistic treatments had worked to rid my body of the disease and to detoxify the dead Lyme as I killed it. I waited for months with baited breath for a sudden relapse, but it never came. Even after the chemical poisoning a year later, Lyme never regained a foothold on me, and I have been free of it for many years now.

Befriending my body was, indeed, the key I needed—I had to change my relationship with my body in order to let it recover. When we fight, we create stress. Stress, in turn, is the main cause of illness. In fighting, our focus is on the negative, the dismantling, the big NO. Mother Teresa is famous for saying she would not attend an anti-war rally but would gladly go to a peace rally. Working toward, rather than working against, is much more powerful a method for everything.

What Are You Fighting Against Right Now?

Whether it's your physical state in general, or an ailment specifically, are you working against something rather than for it? Try feeling into the idea that, if you were to help your body work to be stronger than whatever is ailing you, your body would persevere into wellness. Imagine what it would feel like if your body were your closest friend. What would this mean to you? If it's helpful, pull out your wellness journal and document your thoughts. Feel into what it would be like to have your body as your closest ally and write down those words as truth to power.

Stop the Fight, Begin the Friendship

Spend at least a few minutes feeling into what it would be like to just love your body. A moment at a time, reassure your body that you will get well together. Tell it what an amazing job it has done, staying alive up to this point. You may not be at your best, but you have made it to this moment! Congratulate yourself for that. Getting here, right now, is enormous. Regardless of the hardships, the struggles, the heartaches and anger and diseases, *you are here right now*, and that is incredible. Pat yourself on the back for having made it this far, because you've done something remarkable! Let your body know that you will work *for* it in every way possible. From this point on, you are a unit together; no longer is your body your enemy. It is your best friend, and the three of you—body, mind, and spirit—are going to be inseparable from here on out. Make a pact with yourself to join forces together, reassuring your body that when the urge strikes to blame it for how lousy you feel, you will pause, shift focus, and work with it instead of against it.

How to Keep this Mind-Set

If you've managed to feel into what it would be like to befriend your body, congratulations! If you have not successfully accomplished that yet, repeat the steps above until you at least feel you have achieved a deeper understanding of the idea and it no longer seems foreign. You can repeat these steps once a day, once a week, or every hour until you begin to get a visceral sense of what the acts of loving, appreciating, and working with your body are like. There is no right or wrong answer for how long this process will take you, or how often you should attempt to get there. Just know that when you do, it will be undeniable. Sometimes it happens quickly for people, with very little effort, and sometimes it can feel nearly impossible. Know that every time you try, you are bridging the gap between your mind and your body a little bit, even if you don't feel it yet.

The tools that follow will help you succeed at maintaining a good relationship with your body. A "good relationship" with your body is one in which you are able to view your body as your friend, rather than your enemy. While this is of course helpful in recovering from illness, it's a mind-set that will serve you well beyond getting healthy.

Far too often we are overly critical of our bodies, whether for how they look or for how they function. I gained 20 to 30 pounds of weight with both of my illnesses, and subsequently lost it and returned to my smaller frame once I was well again.

When I am the size I prefer, which comes and goes organically based on my lifestyle, I'm extra grateful and make a clear point to thank my body often for being so in line with the vision my brain has of its ideal state. This relaxed relationship bleeds out into my being more relaxed in life in general, and I notice that when I feel stressed overall, I put stress on how I'm currently looking/what size I am. Every moment is a conscious choice to add stress to or remove it from our lives. Let's choose wisely!

BODY-FRIENDLY TOOLS

GOOD MORNING TO ME

When you first wake up, every day is the most perfect time to get yourself into a body-friendly mode. On becoming conscious, your body and your brain are joining forces together for the day. During those first moments, greet your body as if it is a loved one. You naturally greet family members when you wake up next to them or see them in the kitchen, and if you live alone you naturally greet whomever you first encounter out of the house. Your body shouldn't be any different! Say hello in as loving a way as you can muster . . . and feel free to do that internally if you're worried about loved ones thinking you're too kooky.

HOW ARE YOU?

Once you've greeted your body, do the next thing you'd automatically do in a setting with another human: Ask it how it's doing today. Pay attention to your aches and pains, and as you feel each one, acknowledge it mentally. Rather than, "Oh crap, my joints hurt worse today than yesterday, how terrible," a kinder and productive thought process is "Right now I acknowledge that my joints hurt worse than yesterday. What sounds like the best way to handle this? What wellness tools do I know help alleviate my joint pain? Body, I'm in this with you, and together, we will work to reduce this pain." I understand that this sort of internal conversation does *not* come naturally. It takes work, but it *does* work. The kindness you offer yourself is sensed on a cellular level and you begin your day offering your body assistance, instead of cursing its shortcomings. Does that sound like a better way to start the day?

THE OCCASIONAL CHECK-IN

Throughout the day, check in with your body to offer it a word of encouragement. You can do this randomly and/or whenever a difficult physical feeling comes up. Some things to say either internally or out loud to your body that help you maintain a good friendship with it include:

- I'm so proud of how well you are holding up today.
- This isn't an easy day, and I want to say thank you for trucking on.
- I love you.
- I appreciate you.
- I'm grateful for you.
- I'm grateful this body doesn't feel any worse than it does.
- Thank you for being with me on this journey.
- Thank you for not giving up.
- I'm proud of how far we have come together.
- I love your (insert physical trait of any kind, from the way your eyes sparkle to your posture).

PHYSICAL ATTENTION

Sometimes we need others to care for us, but there is almost always a level of self-care to be done that can make us feel good, too. I don't mean an Instagrammable yoga class or a bath with expensive bath salts, although both of those are wonderful things. I mean simple, caring touch. Caress your arm with your hand; rub your feet if you can reach them; give yourself a big hug; put lotion on your legs in a massaging manner. I don't know anyone who likes to cuddle more than I do, but I recognize the need to give love to my own body, too. In whatever way feels best for you, show your body how much you love it by offering it your physical attention. Not only will this make your body feel more loved and appreciated, and therefore, calm your nervous system, it will build and grow the relationship between your brain and your body.

EVENING CHECK-IN

Bedtime rituals are important for anyone, and even more so for those with chronic conditions who might need supplements to help them sleep or a bath to relax them. When you do your nighttime rituals, check in with your body and see if you can sense anything else it might need. Let it know that you are here to serve its needs, and you are happy to do so.

GOODNIGHT

End the day precisely as you began, by engaging with your body. Say goodnight, and review all of its accomplishments of the day. If that feels difficult because you were in bed all day, it was an accomplishment that you made it through. Every moment of your life has the opportunity to be a success if you look at it right! You did it. You and your body made it through yet another day, and tomorrow, you have the chance to start all over again. What a gift this is—you are still alive! Thank your body for all its efforts and let it know how much you appreciate it. Find anything to consider an accomplishment, no matter how small, and recognize it mentally. You can also write it down in your wellness journal.

You'll be amazed at how much your body did for you today! It spent the whole day breathing your lungs, beating your heart, digesting your food, and much, much more. Our bodies are miracles, and they are the most tangible gifts we will receive in this life. Say goodnight to your body with a proverbial big red ribbon imagined on your forehead. Congratulations! Tomorrow is eager for you guys to join it.

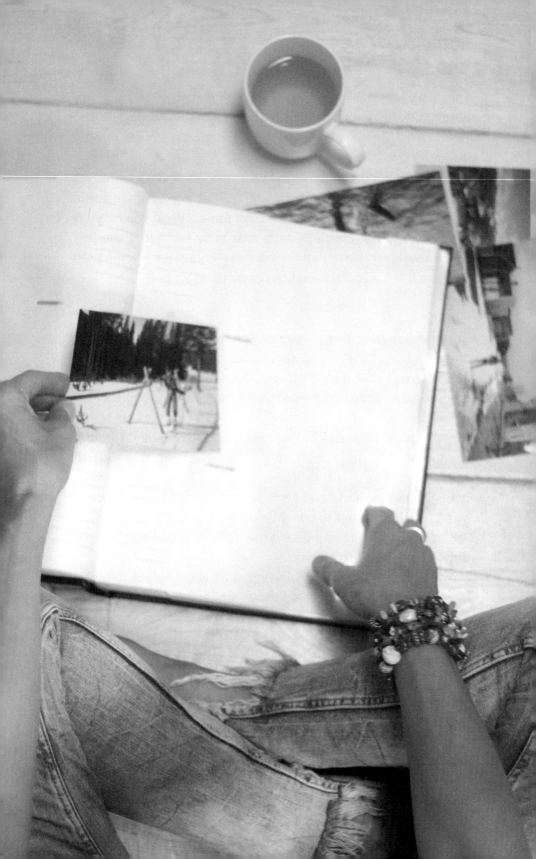

FIVE
Finding the Lessons in Illness

If you share your health situation with others, it's likely that when you do, people will apologize to you for what you're going through. This gesture of sympathy is a natural one; we innately don't want another to suffer, so when we hear that someone is going through a troublesome time, we express our condolences. You probably respond to others with thanks, and maybe a comment about the difficulty of the situation. You may express hope; if that's your perspective, that's a big plus.

My guess, though, is that you don't say that this illness is exactly what you need right now and you're really quite happy for it. Lord knows that when I was sick, those words would never have landed in my mouth, let alone rolled off my tongue! However, it *is* true that my illnesses were exactly what I needed at the time, and I am, really and truly, 100 percent happy they happened.

When I speak about having been sick in interviews, the looks of shock on the faces of the hosts hearing me say that have been pretty intense. Yet every time one expresses their sympathies for my having been through my sicknesses, that's my gut reflex response: I am happy for them, I needed them, and I wouldn't take them back. There is no way I'd be the person I am without having experienced the illnesses I did, and it was through them that I found my life purpose. This isn't a glorified version of the past that I've forced on myself, or some sort of delusional rewrite of history, but rather my understanding that for whatever reasons, those illnesses were the only ways for me to learn the lessons that I was unable to learn in easier, gentler ways.

Does this mean that I'm saying to you that the reason you're sick is so you can find yourself? No, not necessarily. You may already have a profound sense of life purpose, or you may be perfectly content to never find one. I'm not claiming that your illness is inextricably tied to your purpose. It happens to be where I found mine, but we are all unique. What I do believe, however, is that **finding the purpose of our illnesses can lead us onto the road to wellness.**

Slowed Down

In my book *Wake/Sleep*, I refer to self-care as the new busy. We're a people obsessed with cramming in as many activities into our days as possible, and it's taken such a toll on us that we now have to schedule taking care of ourselves. There is a movement to do away with our culture of busyness, and it's one I support fully. It is only through spending time with ourselves in reflection that we can keep what is important in our lives in the foreground. Otherwise, we get caught up endlessly in the day-to-day quest for "survival" from which we may not have the chance to move on until we are too old to do much moving at all.

When you're sick, the pace of your life tends to slow down whether you want it to or not. Sometimes it comes to a screeching halt with you unable to get out of bed for months, and sometimes it just means one or two fewer post-work activities every week. You can see your life slowing down as a big pain in the butt—which, I agree, it is!—but you can simultaneously see it as an opportunity to figure out what you've been missing out on in a personal sense. I believe that when the world forces us to slow down, it means we need to be taking a closer look at our lives and figuring out what we want to change.

Why Me?

There is a sense of self-pity when we hear bad news. "Why is it happening to me?" is a natural question we ask ourselves and/or our loved ones, because when bad things happen, it may feel like life has dealt us an unfair hand of cards. "Why me?" was a question that I got deeply stuck in when I was sick, trying to figure out what I had done wrong to deserve my life going so downhill at what felt like such a young age. Barely 30, Lyme disease made me feel creaky and decrepit, as if my youth had been stolen from me and I'd been catapulted into old age. It was so incredibly unfair that it made me furious regularly.

The truth is that there is no "right" time to get sick any more than there is a "right" person for it to happen to. We may feel others deserve it more because we don't think of them as good people, or that they're old enough for it to not matter anymore, but that's just ego on our parts. We are all made of the same human flesh, and illness can strike any of us at any time. It is not a reflection of your accomplishments or your failures.

Who Were You?

Before moving forward into finding the lessons of your illness, it is important to resolve the two issues above. You don't need to love your ailments or the fact that your life has slowed, but, in order to learn the important lessons the world is trying to teach you through your illness, you do need to reach a level of acceptance.

Everything I learned from being sick, I could have figured out through less dramatic life situations. It would have been awesome if I had, but that's not the truth of my life. While I was a perfectly OK person, I wouldn't by any means say I was amazing—at least not in some significant aspects. As you likely figured out from the preface, there are many ways I still wouldn't say that! I'm content to continue working on myself for the duration of my life, because I think it's a part of why we're here.

It's hard to think about who I was before, because there are so many ways in which illness improved me as a person, but I want to share a few standout changes. That way, you can understand my perspective before we get into some exercises. I understand if you don't like past-me very much after reading them . . . I can't say I'm her biggest fan either.

SKINNY BITCH: Please read this section with caution if you have suffered from disordered eating. I modeled on and off for most of my 20s. When people asked me how I stayed so thin, or what they should do to lose weight, I told them not to eat so much. I had no concept of medical issues that make losing weight difficult, or even of the fact that some people's metabolisms don't work as well as mine did. When I gained weight with Lyme that I couldn't lose no matter what I did (toxins are stored in fat cells, so gaining weight is actually your body protecting you from your illness as well as it can), I finally understood that it wasn't such a cut-and-dried issue. I felt guilty, and ashamed, about all the people I'd told to just eat less, as if that alone would solve all of their weight problems. It was a condescending perspective that likely led to many people feeling crappy about their own bodies and their lack of control over them.

GRAMMAR POLICE: My brain is a sharp one, which is good when it comes to remembering what I need at the grocery store, and bad when the topic is noticing other people's imperfections. I corrected people's grammar often, having no idea that pointing out something that was likely a challenge for another person was a mean act. I thought anyone could learn to do better at any given time, so my corrections should have helped them and they should have responded with thanks. I scoffed at people using mundane words as descriptors, thinking them too lazy to ever pick up a thesaurus and become a better, more interesting person. Then, as Lyme disease ravaged my brain, I lost the bulk of my own vocabulary and had trouble even stringing basic sentences together. I couldn't comprehend many obvious concepts, such as why the 10 freeway ended in Santa Monica, California (because that's where the ocean is!); if I looked at a piece of my writing from years prior, I didn't know what many of the words I'd used before even meant. Suddenly I understood that having great English skills is a gift not everyone shares, and that I had essentially been belittling others and making them feel stupid with my "help."

BEAUTY QUEEN: I spent years getting paid for how I looked. I was a successful commercial model despite being 5'6", tattooed, and ethnically ambiguous, and I was proud of that. However, I looked quite different hunched over with fibromyalgia, sallow skinned, and bloated. I'd always taken being pretty for granted, figuring I'd be many years older before the world stopped treating me specially for my looks. Then, crash, they were gone. I had placed so much value on them, it was hard to feel in any way secure about what else I had to offer as a person—especially with how deteriorated my brain was. I realized why people often appreciate those with good personalities over those with good looks. Who you are inside has so much more meaning, which sounds obvious, but it hadn't been to me.

The Hard Way

Those are just a few examples of who I was before getting sick, and how Lyme disease changed me into a nicer, humbler, much more decent person. I'm sure that I could have learned how to be those things without a life-changing illness, but I didn't. Whatever it takes is whatever it takes! That so many aspects of what had been my identity were taken from me in sickness, meant I had to become someone better in order to be well. The visualization I had in the mirror after therapy referenced in the last chapter was a pivotal moment for me. The process for you might be slower, quicker, or otherwise different.

I've mentioned that after Lyme, I felt like a better human, but I still had no sense of life purpose. I'm convinced that this is why I got chemical poisoning. Lyme *could* have shown me purpose, surely . . . but it didn't. Or, if it did, I remained blind to it. There are so many ways I could have learned from that multi-year illness that food and recovery were the right field for me. People certainly said it often enough to me! I didn't feel it, at least not on any deep level, so I continued wondering why I was on the planet, feeling like I had no reason for being here. Within a year, I was laid up again.

The world tries to teach us gently; I feel confident in that. It hands us small, easy life lessons to learn from. Sometimes, we succeed. Other times, we ignore its attempts wholeheartedly, without realizing there is any opportunity for our own personal growth. So, it goes ahead and bashes us over the head with the lesson, and we take the hard route to become people we like more. I wouldn't go back to the person I was before, for anything! I'd like to think I'm as pretty and as smart as I was before illnesses, only now I'm not so judgmental. And I never, ever correct anyone's grammar, because that's just freaking rude.

Hopefully you now have an understanding of how illness,

by forcing you to slow down and by throwing you out of your comfort zone, gives you a chance to come out the other side a better version of yourself. Let's look at how you can get there on your own.

Timeline

In your wellness journal, write down the activities you currently lack the energy to perform. Track them by day, or by week, or by month, depending on how often you normally did them. Then, add them up; how many hours a day, or week, or month, do you have free now, that you didn't before? This is the amount of time the world is currently giving you to figure out what you need to change about your life. Each time you find yourself stressing over the activity you can't do, guide your mind to think of the time you now have instead. This is a gift. It may be one you want to give back, but because it's been forced upon you, what will you do with it?

If you spend no other time doing the self work that will help you heal, do it during these hours. Do the exercises in this book, meditate, or conduct simple self-care acts such as taking a long bath or reading a good book.

Digging Deeper

You've calculated how much extra time you have, and you know you can use it to help you find the lessons in illness. This next task is a little uncomfortable, but there's no way to get around it: It's time for some self-analysis.

Make a list of attributes about yourself that you have a sense might not be serving you. These are most easily the complaints others in your world have had about you that add up to a theme. If one person has stated you have selfish tendencies, but no one else has ever mentioned it, it's probably not a serious problem.

But if "selfish" is a word you've heard used about yourself more times than you can count, chances are it's worth looking at.

Once you've compiled this list, which can have as few or as many items on it as come to mind without struggle, highlight two or three that seem the most tackle-able to you. Don't start with something that involves a lot of the outside world; for example if you're always late it can be easy to blame that on outside forces. Pick something that you know isn't serving you, but is straightforward. Perhaps you are considered impatient, or overly critical, or intolerant of those who are different.

Next, list three things you could do on a daily basis for one week that might make a dent. For instance, if "selfish" is the quality you'd like to improve upon, you could choose tasks such as letting someone else go first in a situation where you would physically move first, letting someone else speak when you want to speak, and really making a point to listen when someone else is talking rather than planning out your reply. Try those activities for one week, then check back into your journal and see if you feel like you've learned anything. If they didn't make a difference, that might not be the thing to tackle right now. However, if they made your days go more smoothly, and others in your world seemed to enjoy you more, continue doing them.

Whenever you're ready, choose another attribute, construct a similar list of three items, and spend a week on those too. You should do these at a pace that feels comfortable, and amalgamate each task into your daily routine before you move on to the next. Before you know it, you'll be having a profoundly altered experience with the world, because when you behave differently, other people respond differently to you.

Higher Powers

It doesn't matter what you call it: God, the universe, Allah, Jesus, or anything else. Most of us believe there is some greater force out there, and we trust it to some extent. If this just isn't you, and you are a firm atheist, I won't be offended if you skip this part! However, if you consider yourself even a mildly spiritual or religious person, I feel this is valuable.

You've likely heard plenty about releasing and letting go, and have tried meditating, even if not successfully. What I'd like you to do here is basically just listen.

Get into a comfortable position and do some deep breathing until you can feel yourself viscerally becoming calmer. With no intention to say anything, only to listen, open yourself up to the idea that there are guiding forces trying to help you gear your life in the direction that is of utmost good. Imagine what they may look like, and feel like, and finally, what they may sound like. It may be a voice of God, it may be your own voice, or it may be just overwhelming sensations of feelings that translate into words. I've come to refer to my own experiences as "downloads," where I suddenly have information that feels like it has come from a higher power, but it doesn't have specific words to it that my ears heard.

Be open to guidance. Sit and breathe deeply and just listen. It may be that nothing happens—often, nothing does. But occasionally, you will learn something magnificent. If you open yourself up to guidance, it has the best chance of reaching you. The more open you are, the better the chances. Put out the intent that you are ready to learn whatever your illness is trying to teach you, if you are. Say it out loud if you'd like to. Then, sit in silence until you are bored, or until you feel something new.

I can't tell you when you'll begin to feel this power, only that the only way to feel it is to be open to it, and that once you do, it is potent. I tried for years before it happened for me, and sometimes it still doesn't. However, I do know that it's possible, and I know that when you are ready to take in the messages, they will come to you.

8

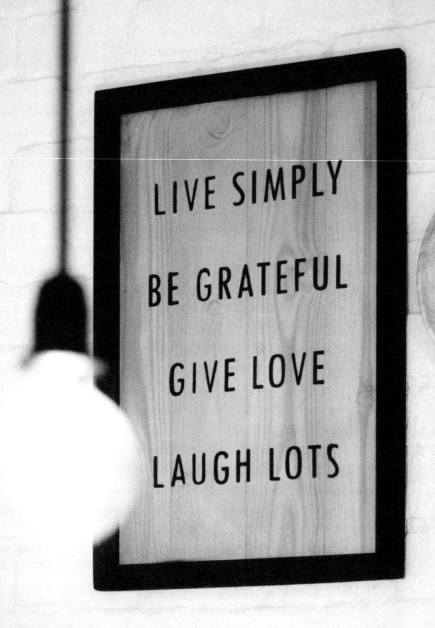

SIX
Gratitude, Dude

grat·i·tude gradəˌt(y)o͞od/ *noun*
1. the quality of being thankful; readiness to show
appreciation for and to return kindness.

It's hard to find a sect of forward-thinking people who don't
espouse the virtues of existing with gratitude. There's good
reason for that: Feeling grateful is one of the easiest ways
to get into a happier mind-set. Gratitude has been shown in
study after study to have a positive impact on everything from
inflammation to anxiety, and personally, I think that it is one
of the most important, if not *the* most important, practices to
cultivate, regardless of how you're physically feeling on any
given day.

No matter how perfectly my life is functioning at any given
time, when I stop focusing on all the things I am thankful for
and instead get wrapped up in whatever is going wrong or
doesn't feel ideal, everything starts backsliding. For example,
I can go from having thousands in savings and raking in the
money from various projects, to flat broke in a month or two,
if I fall into a negative emotional space. I mention this not to
put you into a place of fear, but to display how very real the
effects of gratitude are. Literally nothing else changes in my

life except my focal point. When I do the work—because truly, the work is never, ever done—to get myself back into a grateful state of mind, new projects pop up and my income returns. I've experienced this no less than a dozen times (hate to say, probably quite a few more!) in these five years of purpose-driven freelancing since recovering from illnesses.

It's hard enough to be grateful all the time when you are healthy, so when you're not feeling well, it's all the easier to focus on everything going wrong, and incredibly difficult to remember how much is still right in the world. By entering a state of gratitude, you'll calm your nervous system down and lower your stress hormones, thus facilitating your recovery. Additionally, we'll figure out together how to find gratitude for the things you don't love, too. You've already learned about finding the lessons in illness, so it shouldn't feel like too huge a leap to realize that because illness has brought you important life changes, there are things to be grateful for in there.

This chapter will include a variety of ways you can find the emotional, spiritual, and mental place of gratitude. We'll tackle it from several perspectives because I understand that for one, it's not always that easy to get yourself into a place where you honestly can feel thankful, and for another, what works one time might not work the next.

Keep in mind that no one expects you to forget about your problems and suddenly become Miss Mary Sunshine just because you find things to be grateful for. I think it's vital that we remain real humans, and I'm completely against the idea of forcing away negative thoughts and feelings. I believe that when you are experiencing a negative feeling, the best way to handle it is by actually allowing yourself to be in it. So much time is spent fighting against ourselves needlessly! When you allow yourself to fully feel your feelings, they tend to pass pretty quickly. It's only when we deny them their right to exist that they linger and cloud our perspectives.

That said, the danger of wallowing can't be overstated. Let's explore how to find gratitude for not just the things we love in life, but also for the aspects we have a hard time with, too. I understand that sounds difficult, but promise that it's much easier than you may fear.

Picture It

I consider visualization one of the best things you can do in life, period. There's no shortage of proof that the act of imagining something is so meaningful that your body responds to some extent as if it were real! Studies ranging from having participants mentally play the piano to running in a race have shown that your brain reacts as if you were performing the activity. There is no easier way to get yourself excited for something new than by playing it out in your mind, so we'll look at how to do that.

Each of these exercises can be done repeatedly, and you will have different results each time. The more often you do them, the easier it will be to realize how much you have to live for and how truly lucky you are to be alive.

Granted, I'm Taking for Granted . . .

We all have foundational facets of our life that we take for granted. If you have a roof over your head, food in your fridge, clean water to drink, and clean air to breathe, you are doing a lot better than a majority of people on this planet. We are so accustomed to our first world "basics" that we rarely even consider how fortunate we are to have them.

GRATITUDE TOOLS

Make a list of everything that you don't consider a privilege, but rather a regular part of your life, that someone, somewhere in the world may not have access to. You might want to include things such as:

- Family members: parents, children, siblings, etc.
- A significant other
- Pets
- Heat and air conditioning
- An income source
- Clothing
- A working vehicle
- Education

SENSING YOUR SENSES

Next, let's look at your senses. While you may be having an issue with one or more of them, in all likelihood most are still working, and probably quite well. Make a list of each of your senses (smell, taste, touch, hearing, and vision), and note after each of them at least three items you're grateful they provide for you. My own examples would be:

- Smell: jasmine, baked goods, red wine
- Taste: spicy peppers, toffee stevia, Greek yogurt
- Touch: my pets' fur, the keyboard under my fingers, my hair when ironed
- Hearing: the clinking of ice in a glass, string instruments such as violins and cellos, the "muah" of kisses
- Vision: eyes with soul, phone notifications from people I enjoy, the ever-changing color of my hair

Now, let's break it down even further. Choose just one of the items from each category, and detail out why you like it. You can involve other senses, too, but try to focus on what it is about your choice that most relates to the sense that you use to enjoy it. To extrapolate on my original choices, mine would break down further to:

- Jasmine: its sweetness, the way it makes me think of the tropics, how its smell is so powerful it has the ability to overtake a neighborhood as you're walking
- Greek yogurt: the tang of it that is the exact right amount of tart, its rich mouthfeel that is indulgent like sour cream but healthier, the way it makes me feel satiated
- String instruments: such ethereal sadness in them, how they can be melodious or dissonant, how emotional people look playing them

LESS PERSONAL CATEGORIES

Now that we've explored how to find an array of attributes to be grateful for in things we take for granted and in all that we sense, let's think about general things we enjoy in life, and then go through the same process of getting more specific with them. Write down as many things you love as you can think of, whether they are vitally important or trite, serious or silly, big or small. Some things that I love, off the top of my head, are:

- Colors
- Animals
- Poetry

Pick a category to go in depth about so that you can feel into not only how much you love that specific thing, but how many different versions there are of it for you to love. You can expand on just one sample from each, or list a whole wide array. Based on my choices above, my detailed versions would include:

- Colors: Blue is my favorite color, and there are so many shades of it; I love them all, from baby blue to midnight blue. I also love magenta. The more I think about it, the more I realize there is no bad color at all, and I enjoy the place each of them has in this world. Even often disliked colors such as yellow or orange evoke thoughts of "happy" things like sunshine and sunsets.
- Animals: Cats are my favorite, but I also adore deer, owls, horses, monkeys, and rabbits. And what about unicorns, and dragons, and other mystical creatures? The idea of them deserves my love too!
- Poetry: The way I can help people relate to my feelings by expressing them in similes and metaphors is such magic. I absolutely adore alliteration (see what I did there?!), as well as when poems end with a simple, yet heartfelt short line.

Hopefully, these exercises are making you realize that there are a *lot* of things in this world you care for. The best news here is that you get to experience every single one of them in your brain just by thinking about them! Additionally, chances are that the Internet is at your fingertips—that means you get to see them and/or hear them just by typing their name into a search bar.

Beyond the Paper

On the one hand, I think it's a fabulous idea for you to repeat these exercises as often as possible. On the other, adding a thought process of things you are grateful for is a world-altering tool to just add to the "good morning" and "good night" you're hopefully already saying to yourself. We've already discussed how when you wake up and go to sleep, you can treat your body as a loved one. Once you've checked in with yourself as outlined in the last chapter, and you feel like you are really present inside your body, mentally run through what you're grateful for.

The spiritual teacher Abraham Hicks refers to this as a gratitude "rampage." I like how ferocious that sounds, partially because it conveys the oomph with which you can do it, and partially because a rampage knocks down anything in its path—and that's exactly what you'll be doing here. You're knocking down your negative thoughts and literally running them over into your mind's ground by thinking instead about what you love and enjoy in life.

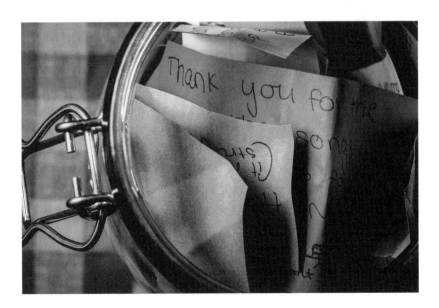

You don't need to go on a long rampage unless you want to; even just calling to mind several items will help your mind-set. You could pick one single category, such as animals or colors, and list as many as you can. You could focus on how lucky you are to have a home with modern conveniences, and list out those, from bathroom sinks to stovetop to washing machine. You could think about how you love fruit, and focus on every kind of melon you've ever seen. There is *no* wrong answer here! What matters is that whatever you're thinking about is something you appreciate. You don't need to have ever encountered it in person. The act of being happy that something exists is completely sufficient.

In the Difficult Times

Once you're in the habit of listing things you're grateful for and feeling happy that they exist, this becomes a valuable tool to use when things are feeling crappy. In a somewhat similar vein to what we talked about in Chapter Five, you have the ability to see the benefit of an occurrence that seems innately bad or wrong. When things go wrong for you in life, rather than focusing on whatever feels lousy, you can find things to be grateful for, which will help the situation improve immediately in your mind.

EXAMPLE 1: You are a having a flare of pain. By default, this basically sucks. You hurt. That means that life doesn't feel as good as when you don't hurt. Seems pretty straightforward . . . so, what is there to be grateful about here? Tons of things!

First, note your pain level on a scale of 1 to 10. Unless it's a 10, in which case you'd probably be in the hospital, you can be grateful it isn't worse than it is. If it's a 4, thank heavens it's not a 5 or above! If it's a 6, thank heavens it's not a 7 or up.

Second, what's your mobility? Most likely, you're not completely paralyzed right now. Let's be grateful for every body part that can still move, even if it's not all of them, because you very well *could* be completely paralyzed. And if you are, is there anything to be grateful for then? Of course: You can still see, or hear, or both. You can still think. You are still alive. This planet is keeping you around because the gifts you have to offer are ones that absolutely no one else can give. We forget that way, way too often, and I'm guilty of it too.

Third, you might be focused on what you can't do today because you're hurting. Flip it around to what you can do. From reading a book to calling a loved one you haven't talked to lately to doing a long, guided meditation, there are still activities you can perform. Thank heavens that even though you hurt, the world has activities available for you!

EXAMPLE 2: Money is tight. Maybe you can't work as much, maybe medical bills are A Thing, maybe your car broke down, or maybe life is just being an expensive pain in the ass. Whatever the reason, financial stress is miserable. What's to be grateful for? Again, so very much!

First, return to the "What we take for granted" basics. OK, you might not have enough money at the moment to cover your new expenses. But do you have a home? Does it have running water? Do you have electricity, a fridge being powered by it, and something in there to eat? If so, you have an amazing life, especially compared to billions of others on this planet right now. If, by chance, you do not have these things, do you have resources? A family member whose home you can go to, or a place of assistance to help you out? As alone as you may feel, there are always forces out there to help.

Second, let's "bigger picture" this. What feels monumental and awful in the moment usually is less of a big deal in the greater scheme of things. Time-wise, let's say it will take you three months to catch up financially from this troublesome

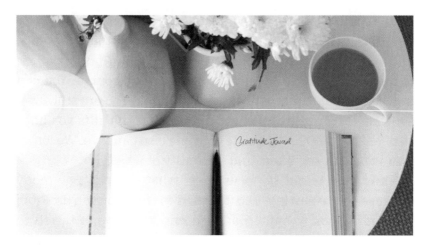

time. That's one quarter of one year . . . and you'll probably live somewhere between 60 and 90 of those. Even if we go with 60, that means this problem that feels giant right now is going to affect $\frac{1}{240}$th of your life. That's about a small fraction of one percent of your life. This feels like everything, but really, it just *isn't*. How wonderful is it that what feels like a large problem is, in reality, only a tiny little part of your life on the whole?

Third, and this will serve as a segue into some visualization talk on a broader scale, one of the best ways to ease your stress about a situation is to picture how great life will be once you've moved past it. This will lighten your sense of how large a problem is, because you can feel into that sense of ease, which is relaxing. When we are relaxed, problems seem smaller. Pause and think for a moment about what it will be like to be more financially free again—even if you don't believe it's possible, go ahead and pretend it is. What's the harm?!?!

Feel into every aspect possible, from what you will do with your days once you have more financial freedom, to where you will go, what you will eat, what you will wear, and any other positive aspects that are pleasant to think about. Sure, this isn't happening at the moment, but it could happen sooner than you think!

Visualizing Your Way There

When I joked to my parents once that in the future I'd pick them up in my private plane, my father said I was delusional. My response was that "delusional" would be thinking I currently have a private plane, because I don't. Imagining having one in the future is in no way unhealthy mentally!

Studies have shown that when we run through physical activities in our minds, we respond neurologically to them as if our bodies were actually physically doing them. This can make for improvement in the activity itself later, when we do it out in the world. You can even increase your strength just by visualizing strengthening exercises. Science has backed visualization leading to real, legitimate progress in countless ways.

If you're finding it hard to be grateful for what you have right now, you can find gratitude in the future instead. While daydreaming might not sound like a tool for wellness, it very much is one. Anything that you can picture that makes you happy is, indeed, a way to help yourself become better. There are no rules for daydreaming; just focus on something that excites you. Feel into it. Write about it in your wellness journal if you're motivated to, or just relish the good feelings while sitting still or going about your day.

My life is one that people are often taken aback by in terms of how little "work" I do to create the life I want. Visualization and meditation are what I credit my success to *far more* than any actual cooking or writing or other "real" work I've done. I visualized this book right into existence by never giving up hope that it would exist. Circumstances lined up for me to write it, and here we are.

You can accomplish anything. I believe in you just like I believe in myself. Dream it, be happy just at the thought of it, and you will help summon it into your life.

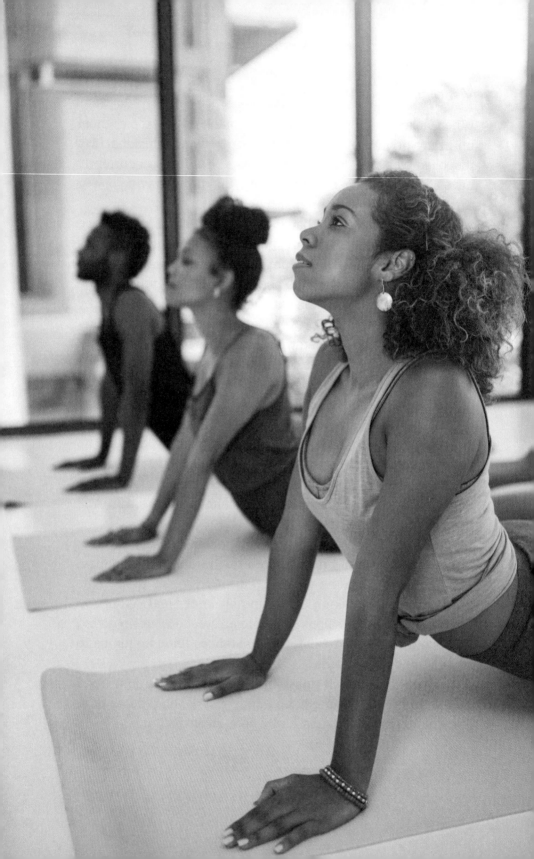

SEVEN
Body Basics

Move It

Let's face it: Motivation to exercise is hard when you feel on top of the world, let alone when you have aches and pains, fatigue, or worse. I'm the opposite of a "plow through it" type of person when it comes to how we treat our bodies. I believe firmly that when all you can do is rest, all you should do is exactly that.

That said, the more you are able to move your body around while not feeling well, the better. This is for so many reasons! Exercise:

- Drains your lymph system, helping to flush toxins out
- Prevents lactic acid buildup in your muscles
- Creates endorphins, a.k.a. feel-good chemicals in your brain
- Keeps your metabolism from slowing further
- Gives you more energy (provided you don't overdo it)
- Reduces risk of additional illnesses

In addition to these concrete and tangible benefits, any form of exercise forces you to be more present in your body. When you're sick, it's waaaay too easy to do everything possible to NOT feel like you're in your body. In situations that involve chronic pain, feeling present in yourself is a huge challenge, because presence equals pain. Our instinct is to do everything possible to not experience the discomfort we are in, from taking pain meds to zoning out watching TV. I'm not saying those things don't have their place; they do. We all deserve peace and escape. However, the only way to recover is to be present in yourself enough to do so.

Whether you're moving a little or a lot, you have to be conscious of your physical self. You become reacquainted with your muscles, your joints, your rhythm. I don't encourage you to start training for a marathon, but I do encourage you to do whatever you can to regain a sense of presence in your physical form so that you can reap the benefits above. Let's look at some ways of working with your body that serve the purpose of healing.

Working Your Breath

You may be surprised that my first, and most important, suggestion for "exercise" doesn't require you to stand up. Neither science nor I can speak enough about the true, legitimate benefits of breathwork. Discussion of this and research on it tends to go hand in hand with that of meditation, showing how it calms the nervous system and rewires the brain. Your breath is not something you control generally, but when you choose to, the benefits are manifold. Breathwork is the basis of yoga, which we'll get into soon, and can be practiced along with yogic postures, known as asanas, or alone. Yogis refer to it as paranayama, but it doesn't matter what you call it; it helps to relieve stress, and if nothing else, that alone will help you to feel better.

There are countless breathing exercises, and they all have benefits. You can begin feeling better without taking on any specific one, though, just by paying attention to your breath and deepening it. This is as simple as can be:

Sit or lay comfortably. Move your attention to your breath; it's something that happens on its own, so paying attention to it isn't an activity we generally perform. Now that you have a sense of how your body is breathing on its own, take control of it for yourself. Take a slightly longer inhalation, and a slightly longer exhalation. Continue this at your own pace, lengthening the duration of your inhales and exhales as quickly or slowly as feels natural and comfortable. Within a few minutes you'll be breathing more deeply. Spend at least one or two minutes at this pace.

Do you notice that you feel different? There's a reason "Take a deep breath" is the suggestion made before any important task. When we breathe more deeply, we send oxygen deeper into our lungs and our cells. We literally oxygenate ourselves better! This alone leads to us feeling more relaxed. Additionally, it's sort of a fake-it-till-you-make-it reaction, just like smiling when you aren't happy. Smiling brings on feelings of happiness when we do it, even if we don't want them. Slowing and deepening our breathing relaxes us, even if we aren't feeling relaxed.

Before going into any complex breathwork, check with your medical professional to ensure it will be purely a healing activity for you. Contraindications to yogic breathing techniques include (but are not limited to) pregnancy and high blood pressure. Once you're sure that this is safe, and you've experienced the relaxation of deep breathing, try one of these exercises. Please note that these are simplified, pared-down versions for the sake of accessibility. If you enjoy the benefits of these breathing exercises, go ahead and do some further research on exact chin positioning, visualizations, etc., so that you get the most reward possible from them. The amount of time to spend is great for an introduction, and they can be lengthened as you get more comfortable and familiar with them.

- **Alternate Nostril Breathing**: This technique is perhaps the most well known, having been popularized by Hillary Clinton in 2016. To do this, you block off one side of your nose with your fingers, and inhale throughout the other side. Then you swap: If you inhaled through the left, you'd exhale through the right. Next, inhale through the same side you exhaled (here, the right), then swap your hand to the other side again, and exhale (here, the left). Continue this pattern of exhaling and inhaling through one side then the other for at least 10 breaths.
- **Cooling Breath**: To perform this exercise, you curl your tongue, as much as possible, into a straw shape. Inhale slowly through your mouth until your lungs are full, then close your mouth and exhale slowly through your nose. Repeat a dozen times.
- **Long Exhale**: The point of this is to exhale for twice as long as you inhale, as the name implies. It's a practice you'll want to employ at night, as it may make you sleepy during the day. To do it, count the length of your inhalation; when you exhale, take twice as long to breathe out fully as you did to breathe in. Try to slow your breathing progressively more as you go, which will aid in your relaxation.

Stretching It to Yoga

As referenced above, breathwork is a big part of yoga. Yoga to many well people feels like the preparation, or warm up, for working out. Because it is always slow in its movements, and because it focuses on stretching, a yoga routine can be very helpful for someone who wants to be in their body and facilitate their healing but cannot perform any serious exercise.

You can look into local classes, online videos, or books and magazines, and you can do anything from one simple asana, or pose, to a complex class. There is a subsect of yoga called "restorative yoga" that focuses specifically on slowness and stillness for the sake of restoring your body. This is the least taxing practice in the yogic world.

Note: Yoga originated in ancient India as a practice that combined mental, physical, and spiritual exercises. It is considered most effective, and most honoring of its origins, to practice all of its elements.

If yoga isn't for you, try to spend at least a few minutes a day doing any light stretching that you can. If moving your entire body is too much, begin by just stretching the parts that are in no, or the least amount of, pain. Move gently, and be kind to yourself. You'll notice that the more often you stretch, the more you will regain your lost flexibility even if you don't feel your health issues are improving yet.

Ideally, you'll stretch your full body, but begin where you can. If only your arms feel functional, do some light arm and hand stretches while lying in bed. Even the act of stretching your fingers has benefits! Any body part that you decompress, create space in, and move around in will help it from stagnating further.

Don't You Wish that You Were a Fish?

If you live near a pool or a natural body of water, putting your body in it is a great way to get yourself moving with minimal injury or risk (provided you don't pretend you're training for competition!). Swimming uses nearly all the muscles in your body, gets your heart pumping faster without putting any impact on your joints,

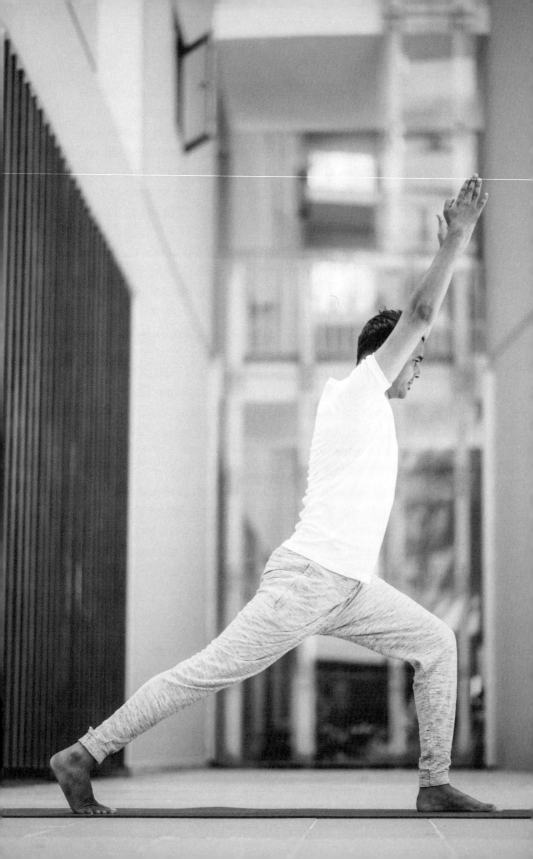

builds your strength, and increases lung capacity, just to name a few of its many benefits. Even if all you do is float and glide around, you'll be accomplishing far more than you would from your couch. Swimming is also an activity that many people find de-stressing, and studies agree that its de-stressing effects are real.

Personally, I find it impossible to feel stressed when in the water. During the summer of 2012, when I had carbon monoxide poisoning and there were very few tasks I could perform with any level of precision, swimming was a godsend for me. My memory was scarcely good enough to keep track of my laps, and my joints hurt like crazy outside of the water, but it provided me so much relief, as well as a way to continually detoxify my body through the lymph drainage that it encourages.

The Importance of Touch

Another way we can get back in touch with our bodies is through conscious touching, by ourselves or with others. We discussed the importance of cultivating a loving relationship with your body in Chapter Four, specifically through actions such as giving yourself a hug or lovingly applying lotion to your limbs. Those are stress-relieving activities that make you more aware of, and conscious in, your body, and there are some additional ones you can do regularly that will further help you grow the feeling of being present and relaxed in your body. These include:

- **Pressure**: Push gently with your hands on the tops of your thighs, the outsides of your arms, or your chest/heart area. Breathe deeply as you do so. This provides a sense of comfort, similar to putting a thunder shirt on a pet. I have unintentionally practiced this myself many a time—during heartbreak situations, I spend a lot of time unconsciously applying pressure to my chest as I read or meditate.

- **Massage**: Lymphatic massage is a healing tool that offers a lot of detoxifying assistance, which is wonderful when your own system is sluggish. It is a gentle form of massage that can feel like you are floating in a body of water with its light, waving motions. If you can't go to a practitioner, you can look up some basic techniques and have a loved one try it on you.
- **Body-focused energy work**: I promised we'd stick to science in this book, so I'm going to keep it real simple here and not go making any woo woo claims that may read to you as endorsement of "snake oil." There are many concrete examples of energy work that focus on your physical body, rather than your etheric one. One example of this is EFT, which is the Emotional Freedom Technique. It's also known as tapping, as you do it by tapping with your fingers on different areas of your body. It holds up well to study. Another example is acupuncture, which involves placing very small needles in areas of your body that, according to Chinese medicine, correspond with organs and energy centers. The ancient practice has been studied copiously in recent years by science and has been proven to help with everything from chronic pain to PTSD, although more research is still needed.

Knowing When to Say When

Fitness experts espouse the importance of rest days in order for your body to be in its best shape on the days when you train; this same principle holds true when looking at less vigorous movement. It's important to allow yourself days of relaxation; it's equally important that when you do take part in activities, you don't overexert yourself. Causing injury will only set back your recovery! Be kind to your body, and remember that this is a time to learn how to listen to what it needs, not beat it into submission. If you're unsure about an activity being the right

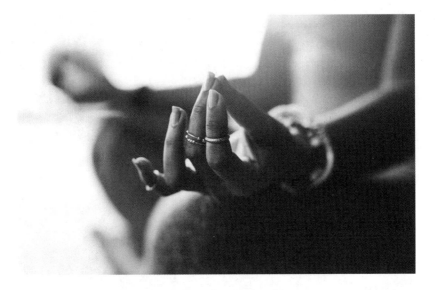

choice for you right now, don't take part until you've thought it over and feel good about it.

Fear vs. Preservation

When it comes to your body right now, there's a chance that you get more confused or overwhelmed than normal about what the "right" thing to do is. If you're unsure about how much movement to take on, focus on separating fear (of making yourself worse, or of trying something new) from the reality of what you are capable of. Are you uncomfortable with tapping because it sounds kooky, or because you really think it won't help? My guess is the former, because before you try something, you have absolutely no way at all of knowing if it will or won't help. I have been surprised countless times by what works and doesn't work for me, and those things change over time, too. Just because you had a less-than-stellar experience with something 20 years ago doesn't mean you will now. An open mind is key here, as is really listening to your inner voice to guide you about what could benefit your body the most.

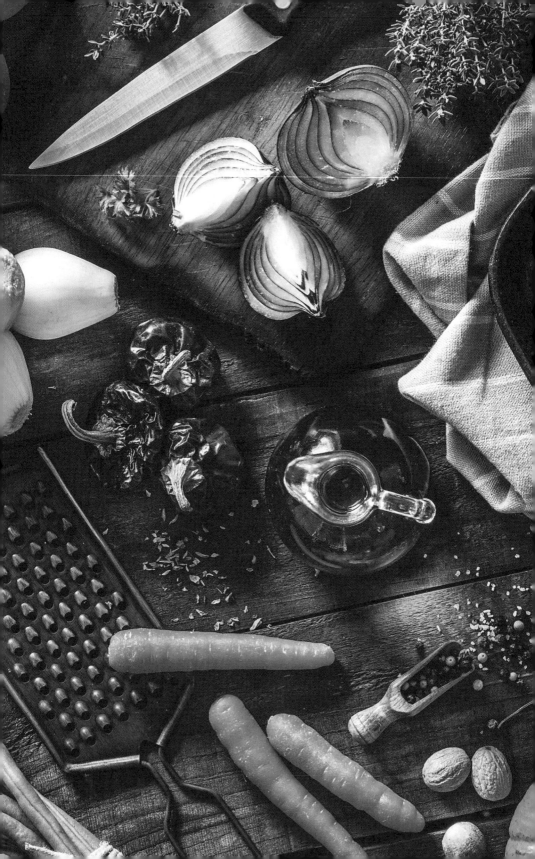

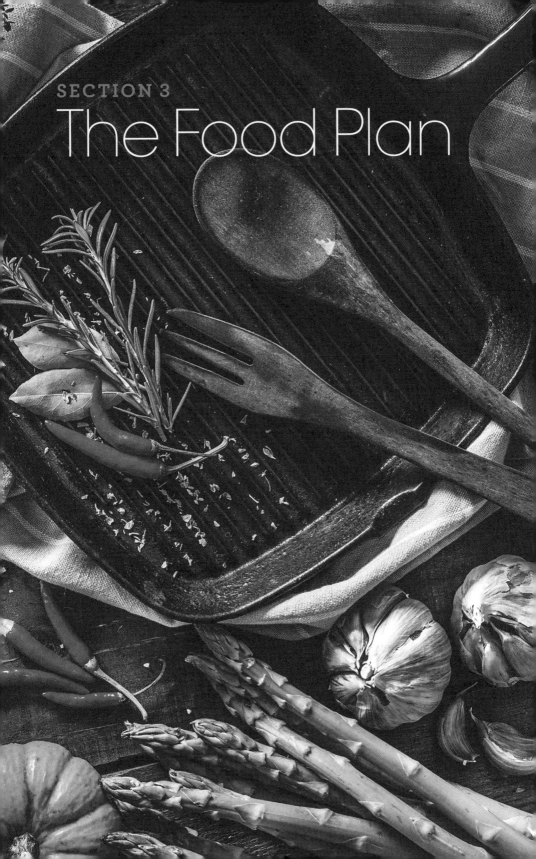

SECTION 3

The Food Plan

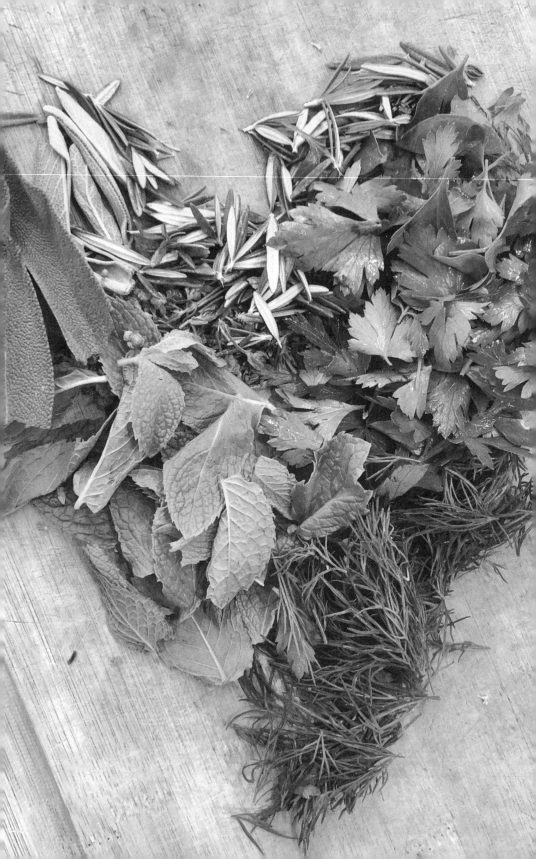

EIGHT
How to Think About Food

Spoiler Alert

This food plan isn't going to tell you exactly what you should and shouldn't be eating, when you should time your meals to be eaten each day, or which diet is the right one for you. As you've probably guessed by now, that all goes pretty against what I stand for as a person and as a nutritionist.

Instead, we're going to talk about how you can best answer the questions above for yourself. You'll be free to make all the choices that feel best for you, without any concern that there's a person out there who gave you advice that you aren't heeding. All of my advice is about doing what feels right to you!

There's a problem with that, I know . . . how are you supposed to know what's right for you?? You're reading this because you want guidance, I get that—but we can take an entirely new route and still arrive where you need to be. I think you're going to like it a lot more than any strict rules to follow.

The "Normal" Way

Typically, when you go to see a nutritionist, they'll tell you which foods work to alleviate the ailment(s) you're experiencing. While this does have a scientific basis, in my experience, all too often the foods that "work" for health issues just aren't properly digested by the people who have those issues. Case in point beyond all else is, tragically, vegetables. The healthiest food group on the planet is also the most complex one on your digestive system, full of myriad types of fiber and sugars that do not always make it through you smoothly.

It is because I kept finding that people were having such issues digesting the foods they thought they were "supposed" to be eating, and in turn making themselves so much worse for the wear, that I changed my coaching approach completely. Not surprisingly, when I was sick I also dealt with not being able to process the foods that I thought would serve me best. Because of all this, my approach is softer, gentler, and more intuition-based.

Step One: Food Feelings

If there's one thing I don't like to do, it's take the fun out of food. For this reason, I've never been into food diaries. Just as weighing your food can suck the joy from it, keeping track of every nibble and bite seems equally tedious.

Conversely, the first step to my food plan only works without recorded notes if you have a fabulous memory. If you do, great! Please, don't write anything down. For everyone else, start keeping track of what you eat—not to count calories, but to discern what's working for you. You don't need to track exact quantities, but do track main ingredients, or any additives (including spices) that you suspect you may be having an issue with.

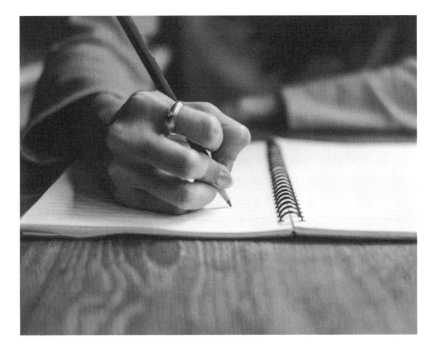

Underneath each meal or snack, write a sentence or two about how you felt immediately after eating. When you go to record the next thing you ate, write more about the previous one, specifically about how you felt in the hours following that meal or snack. Don't worry, this isn't a long-term task! If your diet has any kind of regularity it will take at most a week to get the answers you need about what your food is, or isn't, doing for your healing.

Step Two: Being Your Own Psychic

One sentence that I've spoken more than most others is, "The energy you have about what you eat is as important as what you eat." That's because I believe it deeply, and see it play out endlessly. When you eat, you're no doubt having thoughts and feelings about your food. The work I encourage you to do here is twofold:

First, **be real with yourself about what you're feeling** emotionally. Are you guilty because you're about to eat a doughnut, are you angry because you're eating more &$%&% broccoli, are you senselessly bored with quinoa? Whatever you're feeling is, of course, fine—you're your own human—but you don't want to eat while experiencing negative emotions. I say that not as a woo-woo hippie, but because negative emotions equal stress, and stress equals increased cortisol production. Stress hormones are the hardcore opposite of digestive aids! Negative emotions when eating result in poor digestion.

So, how do you stop this process? Deal with those emotions, and eat once you have. I'm not saying you need a 60-minute guided meditation or anything, just spend however many moments you need to feel good about what you're about to put in your body. If it's a doughnut, realize you're eating it for the sake of joy, and you deserve joy. If it's broccoli and you're not crazy about the taste but you know it's a good choice for your body, thank your body for working better with broccoli inside of it, and be grateful that it does. Or, throw some butter on that broccoli; the vitamins in vegetables are mostly fat-soluble anyway, and need to be eaten with fat to be used by your body. Whatever you need to do to get into a better emotional space before you eat, do that first.

Second, and this is a big one, is **drop the dogma**. I know that is so, so much easier said than done. We are inundated nonstop with "rights" and "wrongs" about what to eat, with conflicting info thrown at us from every direction. I've long since learned that whichever side you want to take in a theoretical food fight, you can probably find at least a handful of studies to back your claims. The "right" answers are forever changing! The deeper we delve, the more we learn, and the more wrong we were a month, a year, or a decade ago. Because of this, you'll be best served by making your own decisions about what's right for you.

When you record how the food you ate made you feel, the main question is whether you responded positively or negatively to the last thing(s) you ate. Some examples of foods that are working for you would be recorded feelings such as:

- Full, but not weighed down
- Energized
- Felt the need to use the bathroom, but without pain or cramping leading up to it
- Alive and vibrant

Some examples of feelings that display your food choices are not serving your body at this time would be:

- Bloated
- Gassy
- Tired
- Over-full
- Lethargic/lazy
- Brain fogged
- Cramping stomach

Each day, before you eat your first meal, review the day prior. Keep in mind what your reactions were the day before so that when and if you eat the same foods again, you can discern if there is a pattern or not.

Sometimes, it isn't necessarily a specific food causing us a problem, but rather, what you are combining it with. If a food that upset your stomach one day doesn't the next, take heed of what you ate it with each time. In general, the fewer foods you eat at once, the easier it is on your body to process them.

Following this process for a week and keeping track of how you're reacting to your foods should help you to find any culprits. I suggest you try life without those foods, no matter how important you think they are, for at least a week or two. If you feel better, give yourself some time before you think about reintroducing them.

I trust that you have your own list of what society has taught you about what's right and wrong to eat, but here is a small sample of the most common dogmatic ideas we are all walking around with at any given moment. NONE of them are doing us a bit of good when we internalize them as stress over what we eat!

- Carbs are the devil.
- Fat makes you fat.
- No one can digest gluten well.
- No amount of sugar in your diet is an OK amount.
- Veganism is the only acceptable diet for the planet.
- Eating animal products is cruel and unnecessary.

Surely you have your own to add . . . I'd encourage you to write them down, but only if it helps you get them out of your system. The truth is that all bodies are different, and there simply IS NOT any one cumulative right answer about what's best for everyone.

When you separate how you actually feel about food from how you think you should feel about it, you'll find that the culinary world has opened up to you a good bit. I'm not saying to eat junk food with abandon, of course; I'm encouraging you to **separate your feelings that you intuitively have about specific foods from how you *think* you should feel about them**, based on input you've internalized from the outside world.

Step Three: You Know Best

You've gotten rid of problem players by noticing when foods repeatedly made you feel lousy and cutting them out, and you've stopped beating yourself up with dogma about ingredients and eating styles. Now what? Now . . . you eat what you want, when you want. I know, that sounds like a joke! But I'm serious. Once you are in touch with how foods make you feel physically and how you feel about them emotionally, it's only natural that you guide yourself to make choices that work better for your body.

I'm trusting that you're not going to go eating "bad" food because the whole point is that you've learned which foods are "good" for you. This is an honors system! You're the only person inside your body, and the only occupant of your mind. The foods that are best for you right now are, without a doubt, the foods that your body feels the best when you eat.

But What If I'm Missing Nutrients?

Chances are, there are some foods you now want to eliminate. Chances are also that one or many of them are foods that are considered important. I hear you! Guess what? You'll be OK for right now. Your body will let you know via cravings when you can eat those foods again, and in the meanwhile, explore foods with similar nutrient profiles that digest differently. A few examples of some swaps you might try are:

- Sweet potatoes: Eat carrots or bell peppers for lutein, or beets for a sweet carb.
- Kale: Eat baby spring mix for a chlorophyll-filled food with less fiber.
- Cabbage: Try sauerkraut or kimchi for a probiotic version.
- Rice: Choose quinoa, millet, or barley for less constipating grains.
- Beef: Branch out to bison or lamb for lower fat content

Those are but a few ideas; whatever it is you can't currently get down well, there is something else out there you likely can.

If there isn't, chances are you will be OK for the short term regardless—the most important thing is to give your body a break from trying to process foods it can't currently process.

My Sick Food Situation

Both times I was sick, my digestion went to pot. There was a period with Lyme disease where I don't recall eating much besides brown rice pasta and salad greens. Was that ideal? Goodness, no! Did it give my body enough to survive on for the brief moment when digesting anything else was impossible? Yes, for sure. I do not, by any means, advocate those two food items become your staples, and they aren't mine in general, but in that moment, it was what worked. Finding what works right now, and allowing yourself to eat that, especially without guilt, is the kindest thing you can do for yourself in terms of food!

Are There Any Real Rules?

You may still expect a list of foods you should or shouldn't eat, or my very strong opinions about specific food items. Sorry, Charlie, but I want this to be all about you getting to know yourself and your needs better. Plus, I trust that you know the basics, such as the facts that sugar and white flour contribute to inflammation and that fruits and veggies help fight cancer. Those things are true, and this book isn't here to beat you over the head with basic nutritional knowledge. I do have my own strong opinions, like that I only ever eat animal products that are organic and pastured, but I'm also smart enough to know that I'm able to do that because I'm in a place of privilege, and you might not be.

There are some simple swaps you can make that I do think are worth recommending, such as trading out canned goods for frozen or jarred. That doesn't cost a lot but is better for you overall. Cans contain aluminum, which is linked to Alz-heimer's, so I only use them for coconut milk—and I only do that because there isn't any other way that pure coconut milk is sold. Vegetables retain more nutrients when frozen instead of canned, and will keep well in the freezer for months. If you only switch out one canned product for jarred, I suggest toma-toes, because their acidity leeches more aluminum from the can into the product.

It's a given that the more toxic you're feeling, the less well you'll respond to eating toxins in foods. It's also a given that most of us do not have the luxury of eating like billionaire hip-sters. Because of this, I encourage you to choose as well as you can, which means as well as you can without stressing your-self out. Getting well is expensive already and adding to your stress by buying food you can't afford is only, as discussed, adding to your stress—which makes it a pretty pointless act.

The thing is, I trust you. I don't know you, but **I trust that if you have taken the time and effort to figure out which foods work best for you in your current state and will therefore help you on your road to wellness, you're going to make the right choices**. Knowing there is a stranger out there rooting for your wellness and trusting you to make the right decisions (food and otherwise!) to facilitate your healing . . . what better dish could I make you than that?

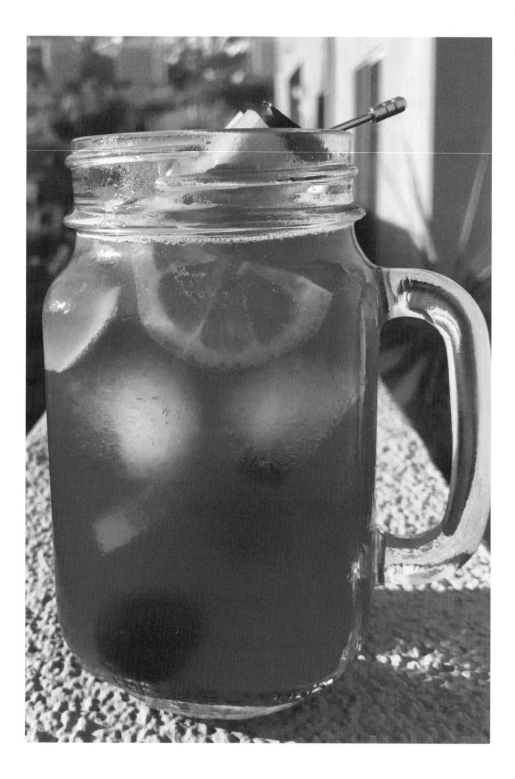

NINE
Easy Elixirs

When not feeling at our best, often some of the suggested food items to eliminate from our diets can be straight up painful. Coffee, tea, alcohol, and soda, I'm looking at all of you! Thankfully I'm looking without longing at the moment, but I've definitely been in a place where it felt incredibly unfair to not be able to have those things. Those beverages all have their places in life, and some offer an array of their own health benefits, but when your system isn't working well, they can be very taxing for your body.

If your system isn't operating at 100 percent, caffeine can contribute to adrenal fatigue; your body's ability to process alcohol can be diminished and lead to horrible hangovers without ever having felt buzzed; and sugary beverages can intensify and worsen inflammation—not to mention sugar is horrible for yeast balance in your gut. If you're not experiencing any problems or issues drinking any of the above, great! You do you, and I'll be the last one to try and pry a coffee mug or wine glass out of your hands. That said, the recipes that follow can *add* to your overall wellness, and they are full of flavors you might be as yet unacquainted with.

There is no liquid more important than water to consume on a frequent basis, but good ole water is far from the most interesting thing to drink. Thankfully, there are a million and one additions to water that can make it even more healthy for you, and more fun! This chapter is a selection of beverages that all have strong health-promoting properties, while at the same time contain enough flavor to titillate your taste buds.

These recipes range from drinks you might want to add to your daily repertoire to ones that are specifically designed for when you're ailing. In most cases, I've left sweetener up to you. I always recommend choosing a natural noncaloric sweetener when possible, but even those can be problematic for some. My personal favorite sweetener for drinks is liquid stevia. You can choose that, or another similar sweetener like monk fruit (a.k.a. lo han or lakanto) or erythritol. If you find that caloric sweeteners work better for your body, mānuka honey is a top choice because it has so many potent benefits, as discussed on page 127 (Cinnamon Mānuka Warmer). Beyond that, regular honey or maple syrup are both perfectly reasonable. I'd avoid cane or beet sugar, because no matter how your body works, those can worsen inflammation and will cancel out the anti-inflammatory effects of recipes constructed to reduce inflammation.

For the most part, these recipes are single serving, but all are fine to batch up so that you have them on hand. There are both hot and cold drinks, and you can warm a cold one or chill a hot one. Also, just because a recipe is cited for a specific use doesn't mean you can't ingest it at other times! For instance, the Cough-Busting Thyme Tea is also great for digestion and bloating, and the Adrenal Restoring Latte is also helpful for immunity.

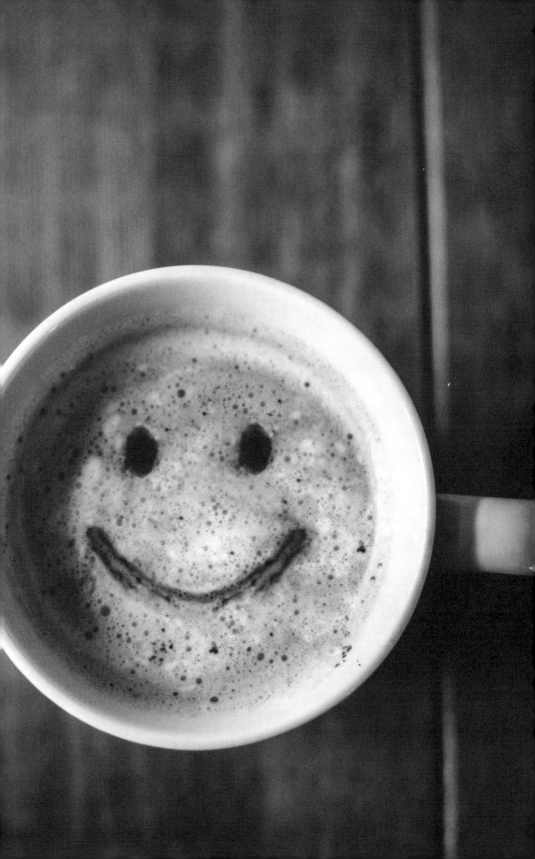

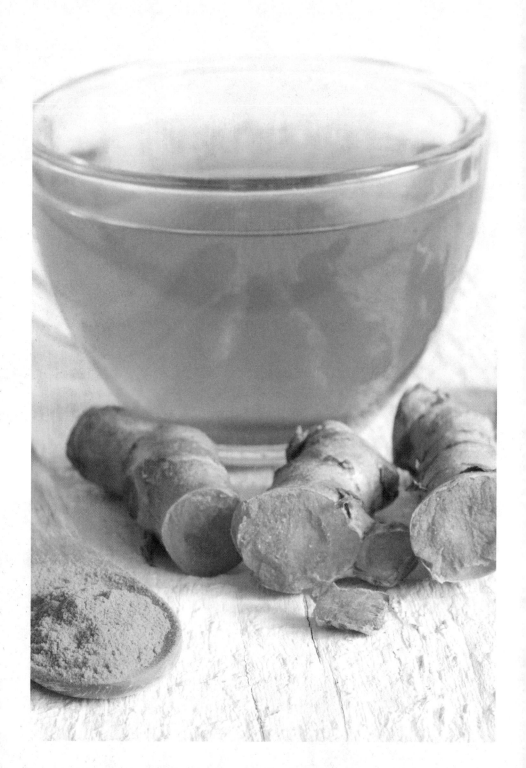

PAIN RELIEF TEA CONCENTRATE

In general, I'm big on avoiding making health claims about foods. That said, I call this tea concentrate a pain-relieving one because turmeric has such solid proof backing its ability to relieve pain, and I've seen it work more times than I can count. The effects are potent. This works best as a concentrate that you can add in small amounts to your water and other beverages throughout the day. The more often you're sending your body the signal to reduce inflammation, the easier—and quicker—that task can be.

Anecdotally, adding this tea concentrate to water and sipping it throughout the day has provided a boost of pain relief within the first week to those I've worked with. That may not be the case for you, but do know that it's possible to feel relief quickly when incorporating this simple tea into your daily routine.

Yield: 8 servings

Ingredients

2 to 3 inches ginger root, sliced lengthwise into several slices
2 to 3 inches turmeric root, sliced lengthwise into several slices
   (if unavailable, substitute 1 teaspoon turmeric powder)
16 ounces filtered water

Instructions

1. Bring all ingredients to a boil in a saucepot; reduce to a simmer.

2. Simmer for 5 minutes, then remove from heat.

3. Discard root slices and store the liquid in a tightly sealed jar in the refrigerator.

PUMPKIN SPICE SIPPER

Pumpkin spice lattes are a fall favorite for many, but health issues can render caffeine taboo for periods of time, so if you're drinking less of it, you may be missing this festive treat. Beyond any issues with coffee itself, the syrup in those lattes is heavily (and I mean really heavily!) sweetened, usually with (low-quality, genetically modified, and very inflammatory) sugar. Pumpkin pie spice is made from an assortment of hard spices, each of which has a solid amount of health value, so let's get them without all that added sugar.

With blood sugar–lowering cinnamon, pumpkin pie spice as a mix has as much health merit as it does warming, holiday-esque flavors. A base of tulsi tea, which contains no caffeine, makes this a healing drink for any time of day.

Yield: 1 serving

Ingredients

½ teaspoon pumpkin pie spice
1 tea bag/serving tulsi tea
Sweetener to taste

Instructions

1. Add spice mix to a teacup and stir to dissolve in very hot water.

2. Add tea bag and fill cup with very hot water.

3. Allow to steep 5 minutes, then remove tea bag and sweeten to taste, if desired.

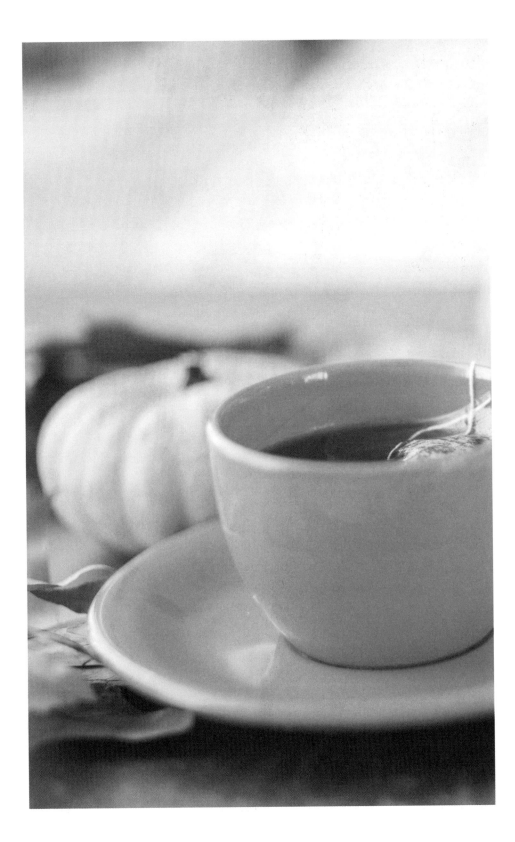

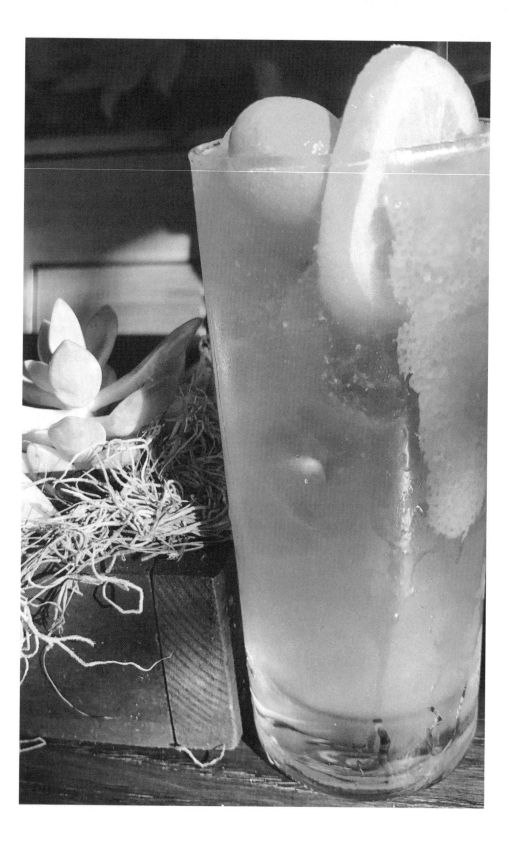

ELECTROLYTE LEMONADE

Lemonade variations know no bounds, but an electrolyte lemonade has a different flavor profile than you may be accustomed to. That's because this drink includes salt, which contributes to electrolyte balancing, and uses maple syrup as the sweetener for its trace minerals (for the same reason). Because of those changes, it's a just a little savory, but the maple syrup also gives it a depth of sweetness. This is a good replacement for sports drinks if you have an inclination for those; if you're going to use it as one, feel free to swap out the water for coconut water, which contains potassium and multiple other electrolytes. That will also yield a sweeter end result. If you aren't using it for physical activity, or if you're sensitive to the effects of sugar, that swap isn't recommended—coconut water naturally contains a good bit of sugar.

Yield: 1 serving

Ingredients

8 ounces filtered cold water
2½ tablespoons freshly squeezed lemon juice
½ teaspoon maple syrup
⅛ teaspoon sea salt

Instructions

Mix all ingredients together in a glass, ensuring salt is dissolved.

SIMPLE MACA HORMONE VITALIZER

This is the fourth book I've written, and I've yet to write one without at least one maca recipe. As you'll see by reading on, in this chapter maca is used twice, both here and in a recipe that is designed in the style of a Bulletproof® version of this beverage. Out of all the adaptogenic herbs out there, maca is the one that I personally feel the benefits of the most in my own body, and that I've witnessed benefit others the most as well. I love it not just because it has the proven ability to help with hormone balancing regardless of gender, but because it can act as a sexual super charger . . . and let's face it, when not feeling great, our sex drives are one of the first things to go! I've paired it here with cinnamon and turmeric; I like how the flavors go together, and those spices are also helpful for hormones.

Yield: 1 serving

Ingredients

1 cup milk (dairy or non)
¼ teaspoon turmeric
¼ teaspoon cinnamon
1 serving maca powder
Sweetener to taste

Instructions

Bring all ingredients to a light simmer in a saucepot, whisking well to combine.

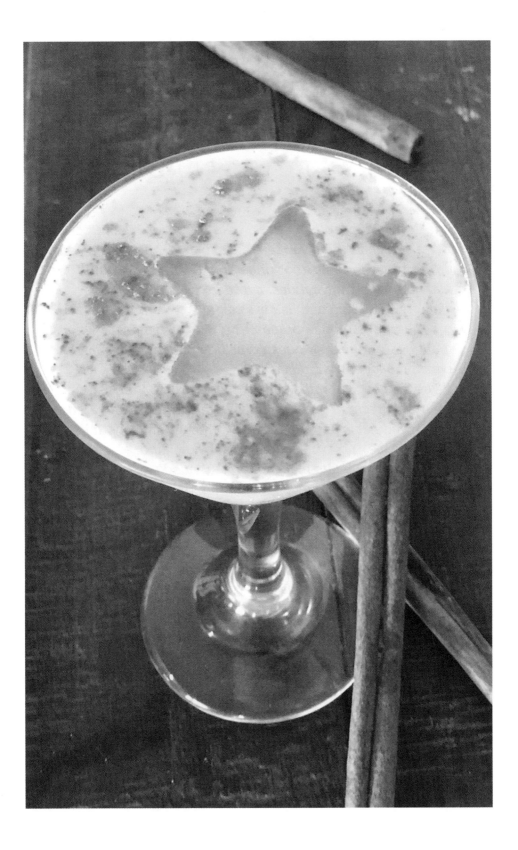

BULLETPROOF MACA HORMONE SUPER VITALIZER (IN THE STYLE OF BULLETPROOF® COFFEE)

This drink's concept is based on the recipe for Bulletproof® coffee, which is when you take a cup of hot coffee and blend it with grass-fed butter or ghee and MCT oil. MCT means medium-chain triglycerides, a form of fat that bypasses the liver for processing and heads straight to your brain for fuel. I use the Bulletproof® brand of MCT oil because it is high quality, fair trade, and doesn't include problematic palm oil (which most other brands do).

The idea of combining coffee, ghee, and MCT oil, as you'll see in this recipe, works equally well for liquids that aren't coffee, and has been popularized in recent times with matcha green tea. It can be done with any hot liquid, even water or broth, and the fats make for an extended slow release of the liquid's nutrients into your system. I'm using the same combo of maca, turmeric, and cinnamon that I use in my other version of this drink (see page 120). That's because the flavors go well together, and all work for hormone balancing. As mentioned in the other version, maca is my go-to adaptogen and I think it's incredibly helpful for energy, virility, and overall lust for life.

Yield: 1 serving

Ingredients

1 cup hot filtered water
¼ teaspoon turmeric
½ teaspoon cinnamon
1 serving maca powder
1 tablespoon grass-fed butter or ghee
½ tablespoon Brain Octane oil
Sweetener to taste

Instructions

Blend all ingredients together until frothy and creamy.

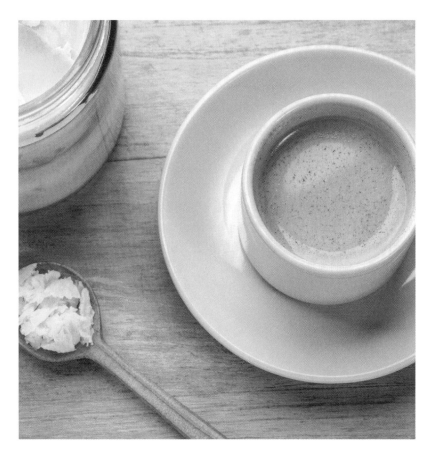

IMMUNITY FIRE CIDER CONCENTRATE (WITHOUT THE WAIT)

Fire Cider is a powerful health tonic that's meant to be consumed by the tablespoon more so than by the glass. Recipes for it will usually have you grate all of the ingredients into a base of apple cider vinegar, then leave it for weeks at room temperature to steep. I wanted to offer a quicker version that would still give you the basic benefits, because sometimes we want to feel better without having to give a month's notice. It won't be as powerful as the original version that sits for ages, but again, you don't have to wait. Like, at all. If you have the time and inclination, and you enjoy the way this version makes you feel, definitely look up the standard way of doing it and give that a go . . . provided you won't forget it's chilling in your cabinet and find it in a year.

Because apple cider vinegar contains probiotics, make sure to follow the step of adding it once the mixture has cooled a bit. Otherwise, that good bacteria may get destroyed by the heat.

Please remember that this is a concentrate, not something to drink a glass of! It's full of potent tastes for potent effects and will not go down smoothly if gulped by the glass.

Yield: 1 serving

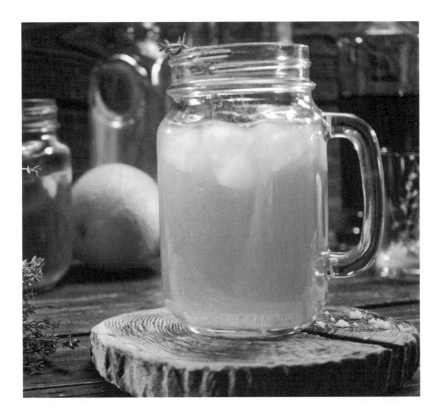

Ingredients

1½ cups filtered water

1 tablespoon minced white, yellow, or sweet onion

1 teaspoon minced garlic

1 pinch cayenne pepper

1 pinch black pepper

Manuka or regular honey to taste

2 tablespoons apple cider vinegar

Instructions

1. Bring all ingredients, except vinegar, to a boil; remove from heat and let steep 10 minutes, until slightly cooled.

2. Strain into a mug and add cider vinegar, stirring to combine.

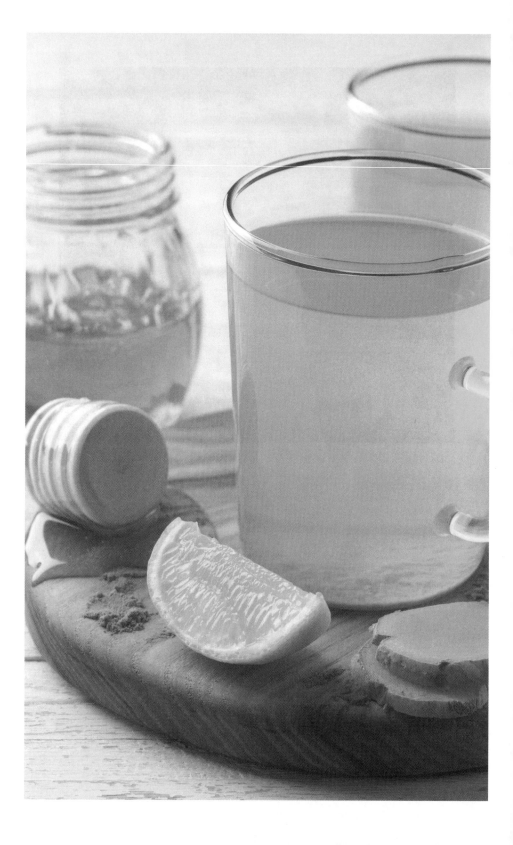

CINNAMON MANUKA WARMER

Once a fringe, or at least alternative, treatment, manuka honey has entered the mainstream in a big way. It's used in the Western medicine world nowadays in everything from gauze patches sold at drugstores to patient treatments in hospitals to prevent infection. It has antibacterial properties that are proving immensely helpful in this age of antibiotic resistance, and is so potently anti-fungal, it's used to cure candida, a.k.a. yeast overgrowth. This is significant because, generally, sugar makes candida worse and can't be eaten by those having problems with it. That you can have a caloric sweetener while helping, rather than worsening, your gut flora is a double blessing, especially if you are experiencing candida-induced sugar cravings.

Because it is still honey and therefore has an impact on blood sugar, it is paired here with cinnamon to help mitigate too much of a sugar spike. Lemon juice provides detoxification and will prevent this from being overly sweet. The result is like a great cup of tea . . . but with no tea needed. (You are, of course, free to use brewed tea instead of hot water.)

Yield: 1 serving

Ingredients

1 cup hot filtered water
1 teaspoon manuka honey
1 tablespoon freshly squeezed lemon juice
½ teaspoon cinnamon

Instructions

Whisk all ingredients together in a mug until well combined.

GREENS TONIC

Few drinks are heralded as health cures as much as green juice. Made of juiced vegetables, often with apple or other fruits added, green juices give you the vitamins and minerals of produce without your body having to do any of the work to break them down. This makes them especially bioavailable, which simply means they're easy for your body to use. Unfortunately, green juice can be hard on your stomach, especially if your digestive system is already sensitive in any way or has been having troubles. I've found that blending produce with water and straining, in addition to being a lot easier than cleaning a juicer, yields a milder drink that is more readily tolerated from a digestion standpoint. I don't use fruit in this drink, which is intentional because fruit sugars ingested without fiber (which you remove when juicing or blending and straining) cause a big blood sugar spike, then crash. This recipe uses fresh herbs that are great for digestion, as well as spinach for chlorophyll and oxygen, and just a squeeze of lemon juice to offset the taste from being too vegetal.

Yield: 1 serving

Ingredients

½ cup loosely packed mint
½ cup loosely packed parsley
½ cup loosely packed spinach
1 tablespoon freshly squeezed lemon juice
1½ cups cold filtered water

Instructions

1. Blend all ingredients on high until no small bits can be seen.

2. Strain through a strainer or nut milk bag into a glass.

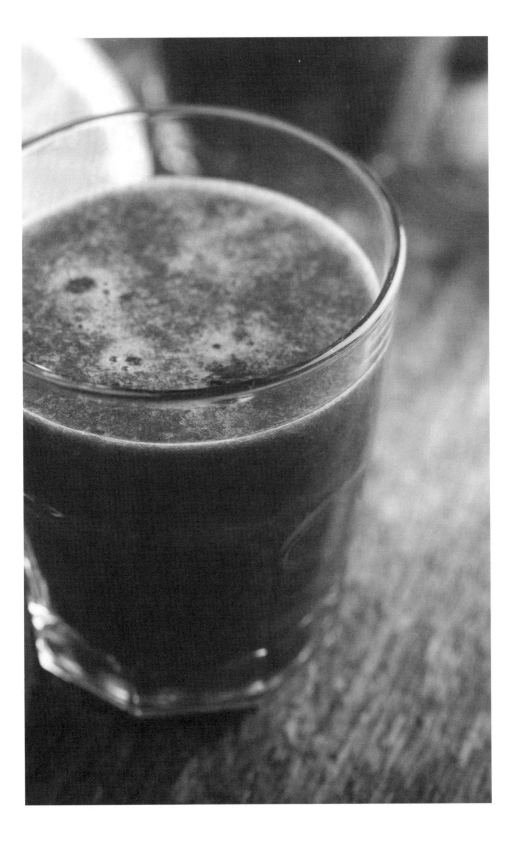

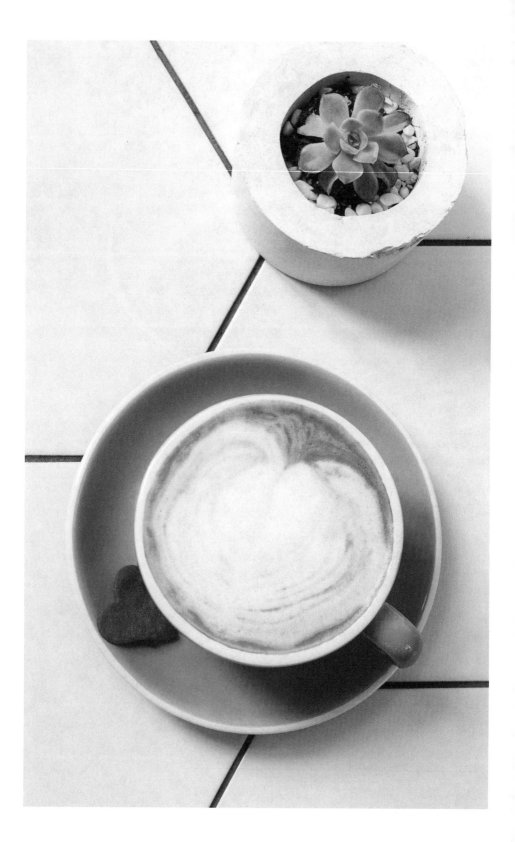

ADRENAL RESTORING LATTE

This recipe is a milder alternative for the maca recipes, because some people prefer a mellow boost compared to a vibrant one. If that's you, and you find yourself sensitive to superfoods of any sort, try this latte first. I've intentionally given the option for two types of tea because they each aid your adrenals. Licorice root does so with added stomach-soothing and antioxidant properties. For medicinal mushrooms, choose any that you know work for you. You can buy them as a complex or individually. If you have decent tolerance for new foods, try a complex, and if you are sensitive, try an individual one such as reishi or lion's mane. Medicinal mushrooms, if used in too large a quantity, can be terribly bitter, but if only a small/single serving is used in a drink, they possess an earthy flavor reminiscent of coffee. They are helpful for your immune and adrenal systems.

Yield: 1 serving

Ingredients

1 cup milk (dairy or non)
1 serving medicinal mushrooms, if available
1 pinch salt
Sweetener to taste
1 serving licorice root or tulsi tea

Instructions

1. Bring all ingredients, except the tea, to a simmer in a saucepot; add tea.

2. Let steep per tea package instructions, then remove tea.

COUGH-DESTROYING THYME TEA

A few years ago, I had a neighbor whose cough was driving me nuts. I could hear it through the walls, and as someone who works from home, the incessant sounds of it was bothering me probably close to half as much as the physical act of it was bothering her. I googled what would best, and most quickly, stop a cough, and stumbled upon countless stories of how well thyme tea works. I went right out to the store, bought a package of thyme, brewed it into tea, and left it on her doorstep with the note: "Drink until gone; it will fix your cough." Brave sentiment, but it worked: Within the day, her cough was gone. When she found out I was the one who had left it, she thought I was the sweetest thing ever, which made me feel terribly guilty because really, I was mostly just annoyed by the sound of her cough. I guess as long as you do a good deed, it doesn't really matter what inspires it?

Ever since then, I throw this tea at anyone I know who is coughing, and it always works, unless someone's cough is from a serious illness or related to smoking. Thyme is inexpensive, always available fresh, full of antioxidants, and it is also helpful for upset stomachs and bloating. In addition to my story, it does indeed hold up to scientific studies as a treatment for a long list of conditions from coughs to candida.

Yield: 4 servings

Ingredients

10 to 12 sprigs fresh thyme
4 cups water (filtered or spring)

Instructions

1. Bring ingredients to a boil in a saucepot; reduce to a simmer.

2. Simmer for 10 minutes, then remove from heat.

3. Discard thyme branches and store leftover tea in a tightly sealed jar in the refrigerator.

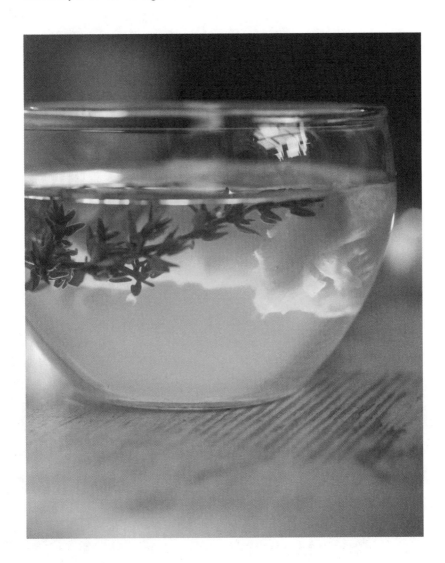

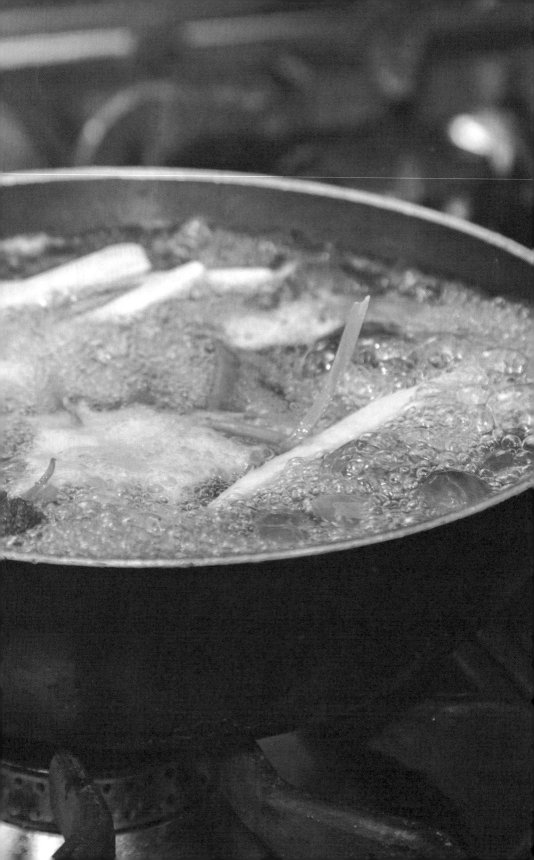

TEN
Simple Soups & Broths

In my previous incarnation, a.k.a. life before I went through chronic illness, I thought soup was the stupidest food in existence. Food is good as it is, so why do you want to add a bunch of water to it?

Then sicknesses happened. Food became, to say the least, a very complex topic that I couldn't escape (because you can't just stop needing to eat). Most things were impossible for me to digest, and often chewing seemed like it would take energy I couldn't afford to expend. Suddenly, I understood soups and broths. All you have to do is swallow, and you are nourished—what a revelation! To be able to reap the benefits of ingredients without taking the time or the energy to chew them endlessly was such an amazing discovery.

Cooking was something else I became a lot less enthused about, as well as a lot less capable of doing. Chopping, which was once so fun to perform meticulously, was a task my fibromyalgia-ridden hands could scarcely tolerate, let alone perform well. Keeping track of multiple pots and pans on the stove and in the oven was more than my brain could cope with. Soups and broths quickly became a go-to.

Not only are the broths and soups in this chapter as effortless to make as possible, they're full of health benefits that go beyond what you would normally get just from cooking some food in water. They're not only crafted to be nourishing and tasty, they should be a treat of drinking and eating, and not only because you're too tired to put anything else in your mouth.*

Rest assured that if you *are* too tired to do more than throw ingredients in a pot with water, let alone to bother chewing, these simple soups and broths won't disappoint you. They are worth the small amount of effort they take, they all keep in the fridge for days, they all freeze well, and they will provide you with sustenance when food seems like more of a bother than you want to contend with.

* Remember, I was a hard sell to begin with, so my standards are ridiculously high for how tasty a soup or broth needs to be in order to be worth making.

BONE BROTH

Of all the healing foods out there, bone broth is the one that has won me over the most. When I was initially in the media as an expert on it, I didn't drink it myself . . . for real. I didn't even eat meat at the time. I had been making it because clients asked me for it repeatedly, and I watched it transform their health over and over. I became an advocate of its soothing nature, its gut-healing gelatin content, and its weight-loss benefits when used as a cleanse.

There is a form of bone broth in nearly every culture on the planet, from Jewish chicken soup to Japanese ramen, and anthropologists have speculated that it's been consumed since we were cavemen. Thanks to epigenetics, which is a sect of science that has shown we carry memories of our ancestors in our DNA, we all have the memory of bone broth as a soothing food, no matter where in the world we come from—what other food could you say that about?! Meat quality is incredibly important here: grass-fed meat is anti-inflammatory versus factory farmed, which is inflammatory—you don't want to boil pesticide- and antibiotic-laden bones, plus grass-fed meat just plain has more of the nutrients you want, such as CLA (Conjugated Linoleic Acid) and ALA (Alpha Lipoic Acid).

The method for this is personal preference: I'm a fan of the pressure cooker, because waiting 24 hours for food, or really anything, is not my style. Pressure cookers are widely available now at a low cost, with the Instant Pot being the most popular aluminum-free option. (I always recommend avoiding aluminum if possible, as studies have shown that it can build up in your system and contribute to illnesses such as Alzheimer's.)

Continued . . .

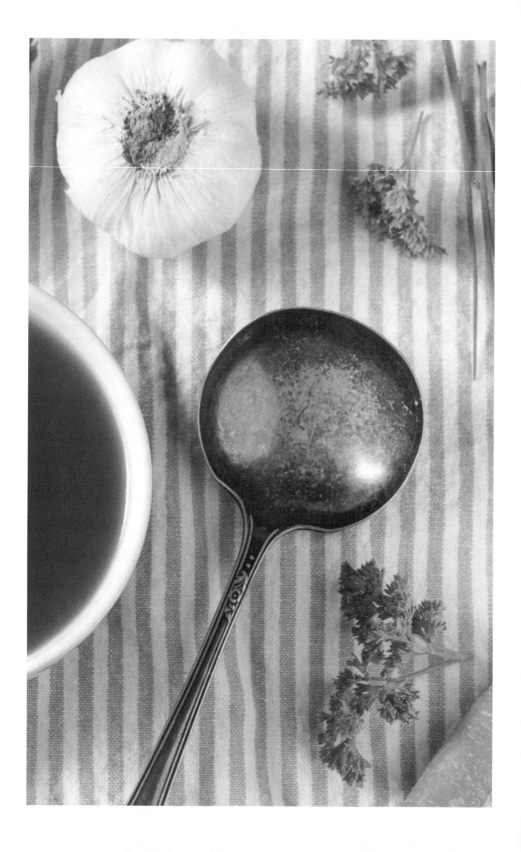

If you do this on the stove, note that I don't personally recommend leaving a gas burner on overnight. If you make it in a slow cooker, be sure the heat stays at a light simmer so that you never enter a bacterial danger zone of too low a temperature.

Yield: 3 servings

Ingredients

1 quart filtered water
1 pound bones, browned in the oven or a cooking vessel
½ to 1 teaspoon salt to taste
1 teaspoon apple cider vinegar, optional

Instructions

Stovetop pressure cooker: Add all ingredients over high heat, close lid, and allow to pressurize. Once pressurized, reduce to low heat and let simmer 1 to 1½ hours. Allow to de-pressurize before opening.

Countertop pressure cooker: Add all ingredients, close lid, and set to high pressure for 60 to 90 minutes. Allow to de-pressurize before opening.

Slow cooker: Add all ingredients, close lid, and turn to high. Cook on high for 8 to 12 hours, or on low for 24 hours.

Stovetop pot: Add all ingredients over high heat and bring to a boil. Reduce to low heat and let simmer at least 4 hours, or up to 24 if supervised.

VEGAN COLLAGEN-BUILDING BROTH

I'm often asked if there is a vegan version of bone broth. The short answer is no, there isn't. The long answer is that yes, you can replicate some of bone broth's effects by using various ingredients that, while of course not the same, can have some of the same results in a more roundabout way by stimulating your body's production abilities. Because the main effects of bone broth are gut healing by way of gelatin, and immunity boosting through other assorted compounds in meat, I've divided the vegan broths into two.

Feel free to throw the ingredients for this collagen-building broth together with the immunity broth if you want this for function over flavor, to get as close as possible to the benefits of bone broth in one single liquid result. These ingredients were chosen mostly for their vitamin C content, which the body uses to form collagen; gelatin is a form of collagen that is integral to hair, skin, nails, and gut health. While bone broth provides you that directly, this broth helps your body produce collagen itself. It has a light, vegetal taste.

Yield: 3 servings

Ingredients

1 quart water (filtered or spring)
2 cups rainbow chard (stems, leaves, or both)
1 cup chopped red bell pepper
½ cup chopped tomato
½ cup chopped sweet potato
1 tablespoon minced garlic
½ to 1 teaspoon salt to taste

Instructions

1. Add all ingredients into a stockpot and bring to a boil, covered.

2. Let simmer for 30 minutes.

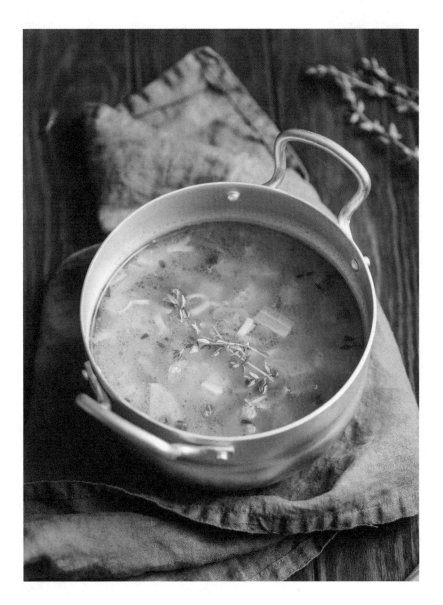

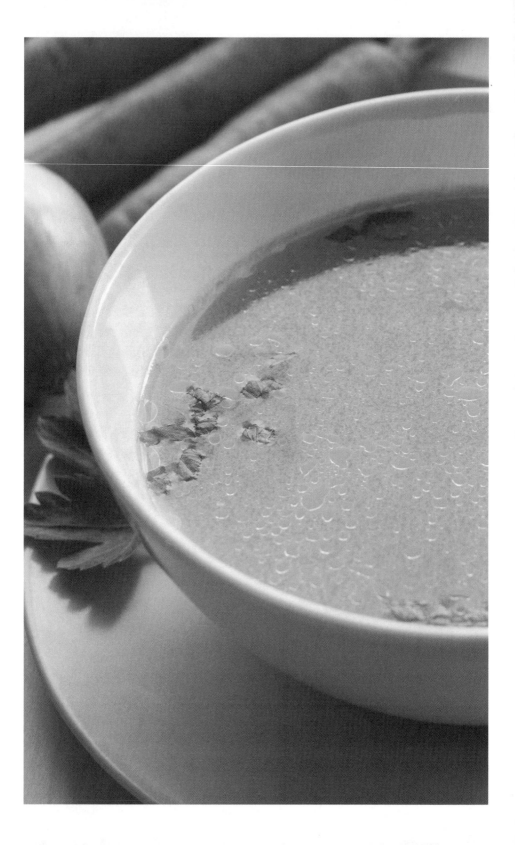

VEGAN MUSHROOM IMMUNITY MINERAL BROTH

Generally, vegan versions of bone broth that focus on immunity boosting have a huge quantity of ingredients. Because I want you to actually make the recipes in this book, and without feeling overwhelmed by the work of them, this recipe is an example of where I pared down things to go as simple and, er, bare bones as possible. (Only, you know, without the bones in this case.) There are many mushrooms that have medicinal effects besides shiitakes, but shiitakes are the least expensive and most readily available commercially. If you have access to maiitakes or other medicinal mushrooms, please sub out those as you see fit, as it will make the broth more powerful. If by chance you can't find shiitakes locally, you can purchase them dried online. Kombu, a.k.a. kelp, is used here both to enrich the flavor and add to thyroid-boosting iodine and other minerals.

Yield: 6 servings

Ingredients

4 cups filtered water
3 cups chopped shiitake mushrooms
½ teaspoon salt
One 4-inch piece kombu/kelp

Instructions

1. In a saucepot, bring all ingredients, except kombu/kelp, to a boil over medium-high heat.

2. Reduce to a simmer and add kombu/kelp.

3. Simmer for approximately 20 minutes.

MISO MAGIC SOUP

When people ask me what brand of probiotics I recommend, my first answers are always foods. I'm a fan of, wherever possible, getting what you need from what you eat before taking supplements. Studies vary on how much of any given capsule your body can actually use, but logic dictates that whatever the amount is, it will be based on how well your digestive system is functioning at the time. Miso is one of many ways to add more probiotics directly into your diet without popping a pill—you just have to make sure to not boil it, or you'll murder the beneficial bacteria. Miso is traditionally made by fermenting soybeans, but is also available now made from other legumes and grains, such as chickpeas or barley. One small container will last a very long time because you use so little at once, so I recommend choosing a high-quality one for a couple of dollars more if that's possible for you. This recipe is a very simplified version of what you would enjoy at a Japanese restaurant. For the heartiest taste, use bone broth.

Yield: 1 serving

Ingredients

1 teaspoon mellow white miso paste
1½ cups broth (bone, mushroom, or veggie)
2 tablespoons torn nori
1 tablespoon thinly sliced scallions

Instructions

1. Whisk miso paste into broth over low heat, until desired level of heat is reached, taking care not to boil.

2. Remove from heat and add nori and scallion.

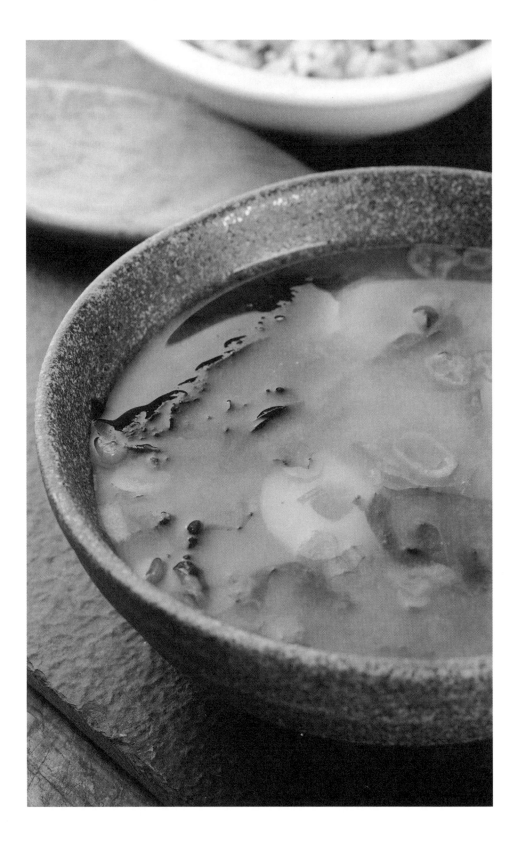

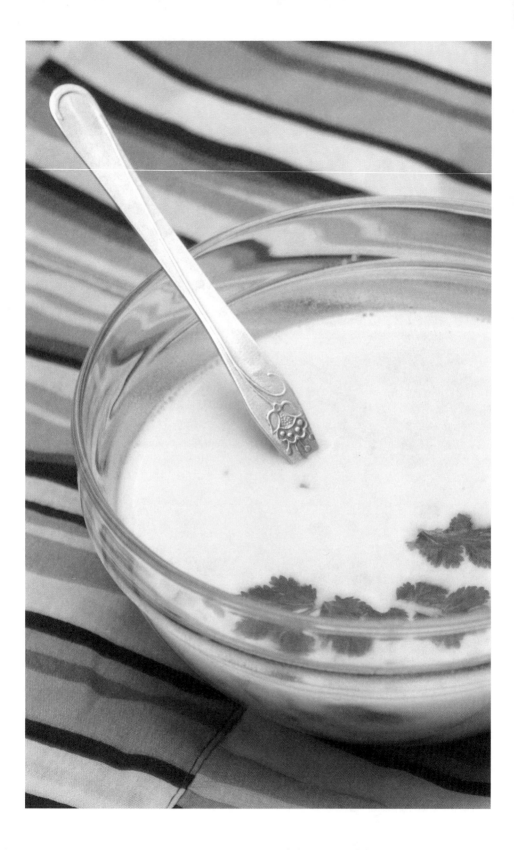

COCONUT LEMONGRASS BROTH

Popular in Eastern cultures, lemongrass is a powerful, cost-effective flavoring that is underused in Western cuisine. It has, as you may guess, a grassy and lemony aroma and taste. Lemongrass is also used for metabolism, digestion, and immunity. Pairing it with coconut milk makes for a rich broth that is a perfect soup base to which you can add seafood, poultry, and/or veggies. Coconut milk, in this case, should be the thick type made with actual ground coconut meat; the boxed version that is mostly water won't provide any thickness, or even much coconut flavor. Coconut is also helpful for immunity, as well as being anti-inflammatory.

Yield: 1 serving

Ingredients

1 cup broth (bone, mushroom, or veggie)
½ cup pure full-fat coconut milk
One 4-inch piece lemongrass
1 small pinch salt
1 pinch cayenne, optional

Instructions

1. Bring all ingredients to simmer in a saucepot, and let simmer 10 minutes.

2. Remove lemongrass.

BEET BLOOD CLEANSER

The concept of this is similar to the Greens Tonic in the Easy Elixirs chapter: Rather than juicing an item, you blend and strain it. That makes for a milder end result, because powerful ingredients such as beets can cause flushing. It is a good choice for anyone feeling sensitive. The pigment that colors beets is called betaxanthin, and it has been shown to have strong anti-inflammatory and antioxidant properties. What makes beets good for your blood is their nitrate content, which benefits your heart's functioning and your circulation. This means that they can lower your blood pressure, which is wonderful . . . but also something that's important to be aware of if you already have low blood pressure to begin with. If you have any issues with blood pressure, I suggest avoiding beet juice and other concentrated forms of beets.

Yield: 1 serving

Ingredients

1 cup filtered water
½ cup diced beets
1 tablespoon freshly squeezed lemon juice
1 pinch cayenne

Instructions

1. Blend all ingredients on high until no small bits can be seen.

2. Strain through a strainer or nut milk bag into a glass. If desired, heat on the stove until warm.

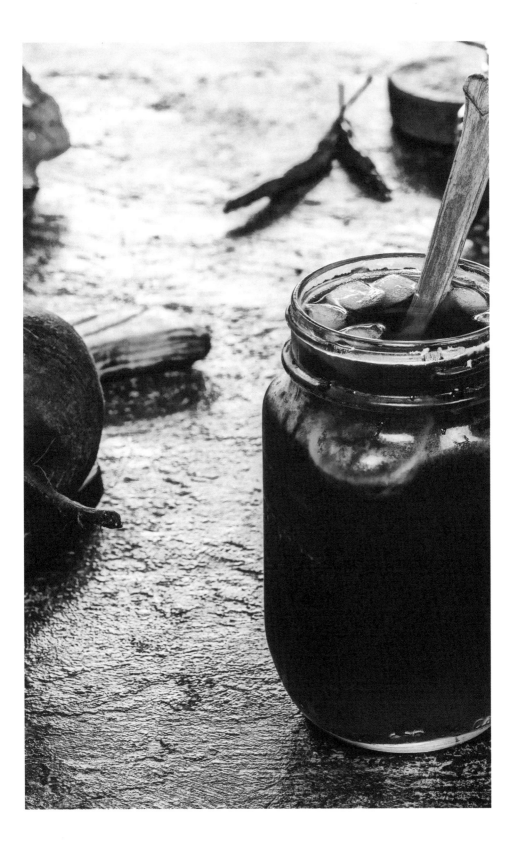

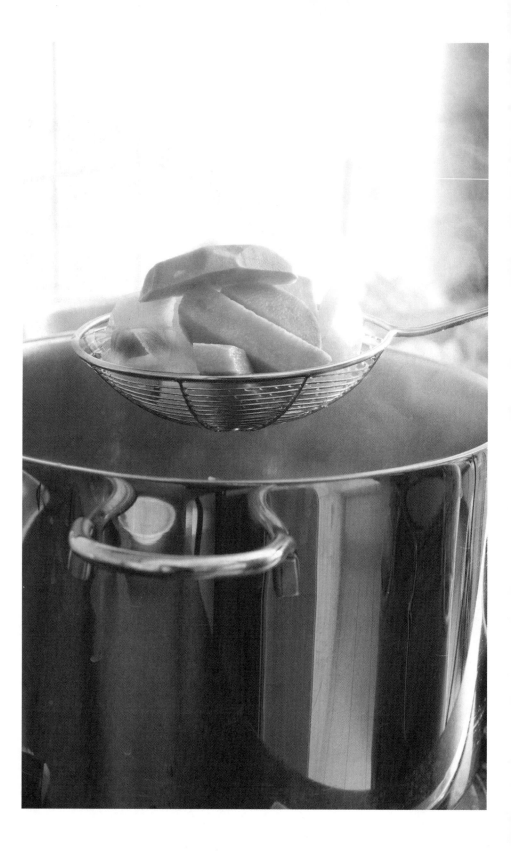

SWEET POTATO WATER

The idea of boiling a vegetable and drinking the leftover water, rather than eating the vegetable itself, might seem a little weird. You can, of course, eat the sweet potatoes from this recipe; they just aren't the point of it. Sweet potato water has been studied at length in recent years for its effects on weight loss and leptin resistance; leptin plays a vital role in blood sugar, and when you become resistant to the effects of it, diabetes often follows. Sweet potato water has also been shown to markedly reduce cholesterol. This recipe is light and sweet, and you could add pumpkin pie spices and some vanilla if you wanted to turn it into a dessert-style beverage. While the idea has been around for a while, it's still growing in notoriety, and definitely hasn't hit the mainstream yet. When it does, we can probably expect packaged sweet potato water on shelves next to coconut, maple, and watermelon waters!

Yield: 1 serving

Ingredients

2 cups chopped sweet potatoes
2 cups filtered water

Instructions

1. Bring ingredients to a boil, then reduce to a simmer.

2. Simmer until sweet potatoes are soft, 7 to 8 minutes.

3. Strain water into a large glass, reserving sweet potatoes for another use.

AROMATIC HERB BROTH

When I was sick, not being able to digest raw, or often even cooked, veggies, was one of the saddest things for me in relation to food. I craved the feeling of eating vibrant, green, life-filled food so badly, but my stomach rejected it with equal vehemence. For the times when you are experiencing a similar craving, this broth will satisfy, or at least put a dent in, your need for green. For this recipe, you can use any fresh herb(s) you enjoy, and it will give you a little bit of that bright, alive feel of consuming greens, without actually doing so. All fresh herbs have excellent value for your health, so choose the ones you enjoy best, and vary them when you want a change. My favorite here is a combo of parsley, dill, and thyme. For the most vegetal flavor, choose the Vegan Collagen-Building Broth (see page 140) as the base.

Yield: 1 serving

Ingredients

1½ cups broth (bone, mushroom, or veggie)
½ cup fresh herb leaves

Instructions

1. Heat broth until simmering.

2. Remove from heat and add herbs. Let steep for 10 minutes, then strain into a large mug.

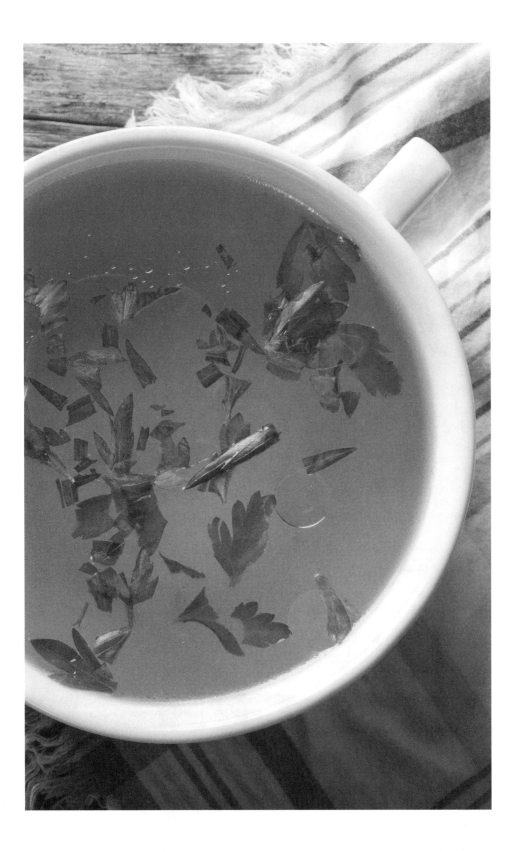

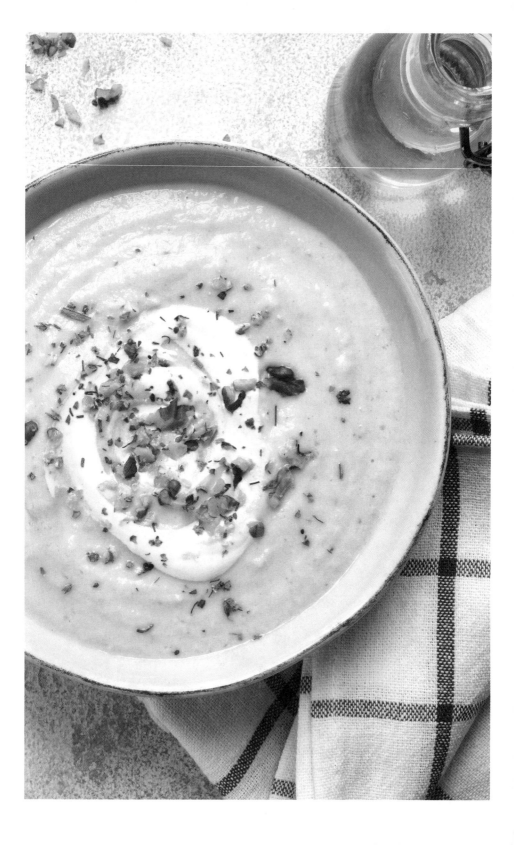

CREAMY GARLIC SOUP

Garlic is well known for its immunity-boosting effects and for being antibacterial. It's most powerful when consumed raw, but unfortunately, that can lead to major digestive upset if your stomach is at all sensitive. Stomach upset is completely outside of the issue of the so-called "garlic breath" that can stick with you for many hours after eating garlic raw, which is another reason some people avoid it. While I'm a fan of raw garlic where appropriate, I also recognize the desire to obtain its benefits in a gentler way—this recipe is a representation of that idea. It is very creamy for containing no dairy, which is made possible via cashews, the vegan world's favorite nut. Cashews are high in minerals, offering not only texture, but also function, to this soup. You'll be surprised at how rich and filling this broth is!

Yield: 1 serving

Ingredients

1½ cups broth (bone, mushroom, or veggie)
2 tablespoons raw cashews
½ tablespoon minced garlic
1 pinch salt
Several grinds of black pepper

Instructions

1. Bring ingredients to a boil in a small saucepot over medium-high heat, then reduce to a simmer; let simmer 15 minutes.

2. Place mixture into a blender and blend until completely smooth.

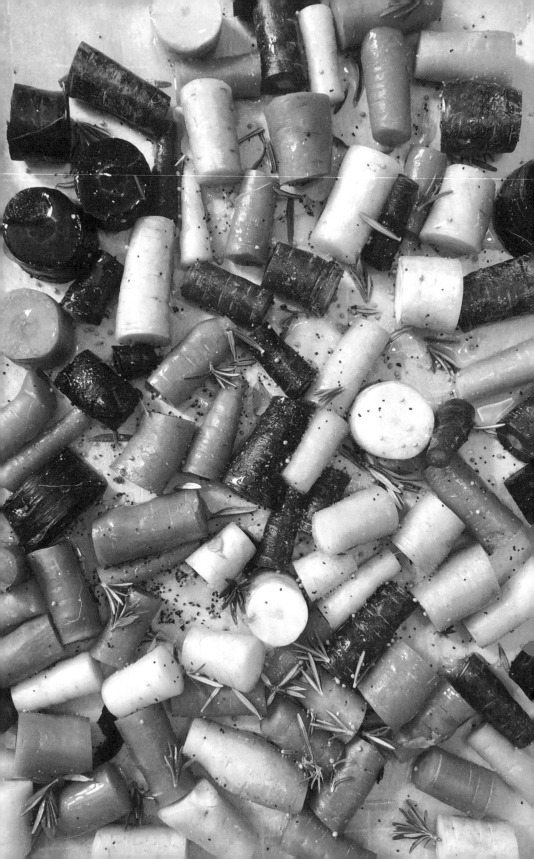

ELEVEN
Making Vegetables More Digestible

You've probably come across more than enough recipes for vegetable dishes to last you a lifetime, and may even be surprised I've dedicated an entire chapter to them, as I've talked so much about how in times of physical distress they can be hard for your body to process. The reason for my adding to the world's swath of veggie recipes already in existence is that finding ones *that go down easily when you aren't feeling your best* can be a bit of a daunting task. While vegetables have the nutrients you need to feel better, they come equipped with all kinds of properties, such as insoluble fiber, that can make it very difficult for your body to process them properly.

When your digestive system isn't at its peak, this can translate into extreme discomfort. I can't count how many nutrition consults I've done in which clients have told me they are eating large quantities of vegetables because they feel like they should—and they are also experiencing major gas, bloating, and stomach pain after every meal. We are so socially conditioned to think that we have to eat things because they are good for us, we've forgotten to listen to our bodies shouting loud, with deafening cues, to behave differently.

The point of this chapter is to offer you alternatives to the way you're currently eating your veggies. The focus is less on straight green salads or steamed broccoli, and more on getting the feeling of eating healthful, fresh foods in ways that won't tax or further strain your digestive system. The recipes focus on cooking temperature, marinating methods, and breaking down the produce. These aren't for the sake of culinary technique, but rather are employed to make each dish as easy for you to digest as possible.

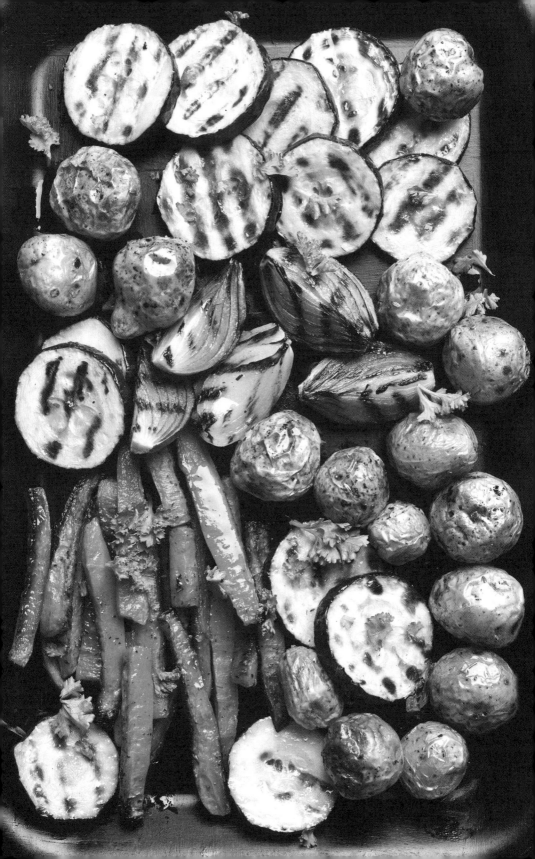

CIDER VINEGAR CUCUMBER SALAD

A refreshing and tangy salad can be a joyful snack or a palate-cleansing side dish, but not if you're reminded of it in negative ways for hours after you eat it! By letting cider vinegar soften cucumbers, you're getting the probiotic benefits of the vinegar that help facilitate digestion, as well as cucumbers that require less work for your digestive system to break down because of the easier texture. Basically, you're enlisting the vinegar to do some preliminary work for you, and to make your body's job less laborious. Cucumber and dill are a classic flavor combo (think dill pickles), aided further by dill having carminative (anti-gas) effects. Cucumbers are a hydrating food, meaning they contain a good proportion of water, that can help you feel full without adding many calories to your day. Because this little salad can aid with digestion, it makes a nice palate refresher between dinner courses or a small bite at the end of a meal.

Yield: 2 servings

Ingredients

1 cup cucumber, seeds removed, sliced as thinly as possible
2 tablespoons apple cider vinegar
1 tablespoon extra virgin olive oil
½ teaspoon dried dill
1 pinch salt

Instructions

Combine all ingredients in a mixing bowl, tossing well to coat cucumber. Refrigerate up to several days.

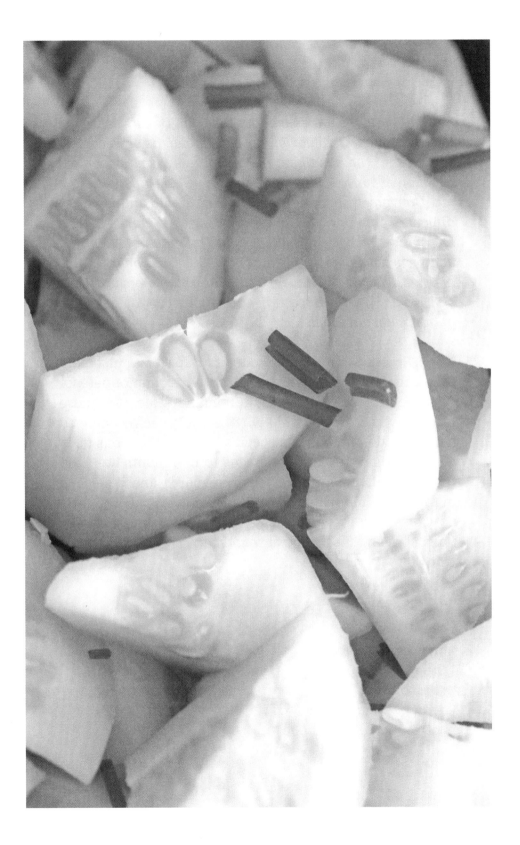

EGGPLANT MASH

Mashed potatoes are delish, but they don't really offer up a ton of nutrition. Cauliflower mash has been the new mashed potatoes for the health food world for a few years now, but cauliflower can be harsh on your stomach, as crucifers often are. Conversely, eggplant has vital nutrients and is not so difficult to break down as cauliflower, so it makes a good alternative to that alternative. If you tolerate potatoes well and want to make them healthier, do a 50/50 combo of this dish with mashed potatoes; that will lighten them up, while still leaving you feeling as full and satisfied as you'd hope to get from a potato mash.

Note: Eggplant is a nightshade (as is paprika, also contained in this recipe), which means it is not appropriate for those on protocols such as AutoImmune Paleo. (For those readers who are wondering why I would even recommend a nightshade in the first place, it's because there has been no study that proves nightshades to be inflammatory, all reports of inflammation from them are purely anecdotal, and in the many, many people with whom I've worked, I have not personally ever witnessed any difference in inflammation between those who eat nightshade veggies and those who don't.)

Yield: 4 servings

Ingredients

1 large eggplant, cut in half lengthwise
1 tablespoon neutral oil, such as avocado or grape seed
½ teaspoon salt
½ teaspoon smoked paprika
½ tablespoon ghee or butter

Instructions

1. Preheat oven to 375°F.

2. Place eggplant, cut side down, on a lined baking sheet that has been drizzled with half the neutral oil and half the salt. Drizzle skin with remaining oil, reserving remaining salt.

3. Roast until wrinkled and soft when poked, about 40 minutes. Let cool slightly.

4. Scrape out insides of eggplant into a bowl, discarding skin.

5. Add remaining salt, smoked paprika, and ghee or butter, and mash with a fork. For a more creamy texture, puree in food processor or blender.

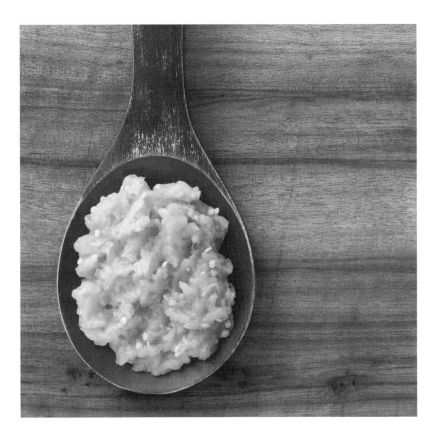

GREEN GODDESS PUREE

This is one of those dishes that reads as much more than the sum of its parts. It has a twofold purpose: On the one hand, it's a hardy replacement for mashed potatoes, and on the other, it has a fresh, green look and flavor that provides you with some much-needed chlorophyll in an easy-to-digest context. Similar to the herbed broth, it can help satiate cravings for leafy greens at times when your stomach is saying no to them.

Celery root, a.k.a. celeriac, is one of my favorite vegetables, but most people never buy it, or even can recognize it. It's inexpensive, it's quite creamy when blended, and it lends a surprisingly delicious, restaurant taste to any dish. It's high in potassium and vitamin K, too. Fennel can be an acquired taste due to its licorice notes being polarizing to many, so rest assured that it's very mellow here and won't make the dish reminiscent of licorice. Feel free to swap out baby spinach for another tender/soft baby green if there's a different one you prefer. Arugula would add some spice, as well as nourishment for your digestive tract.

Yield: 3 servings

Ingredients

1 cup chopped fennel, ½-inch-thick slices
1 cup chopped celery root, ¾-inch cubes
1 cup bone broth or vegan immunity broth or stock
½ tablespoon minced garlic
¼ to ½ teaspoon salt, depending on salinity of broth
1 cup baby spinach
½ cup fennel fronds
½ tablespoon butter
½ teaspoon black pepper

Instructions

1. Add fennel through salt into a saucepot. Cover and bring to a boil.

2. Reduce to a simmer and cook, covered, until fennel and celeriac are soft, 8 to 10 minutes.

3. Place remaining ingredients into a blender and add veggie mix into it.

4. Blend until smooth and creamy or leave bits of texture if preferred.

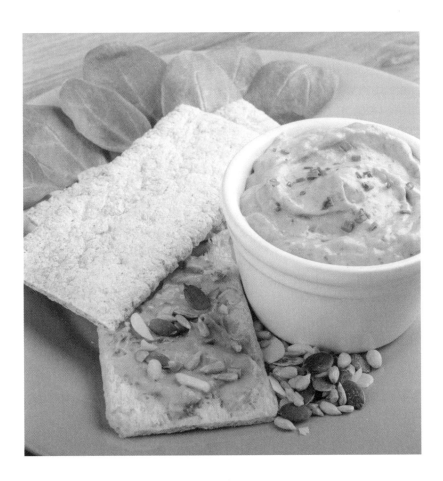

CARROT ZOODLES

"Zoodles" are the term for spiralized vegetables made in the shape of noodles. The z is for zucchini, because that was the main item used when the dish first hit the mainstream, but the word zoodle is now generally the name for that preparation no matter which veggie you choose. While zucchini is wonderful, it can be hard to digest, and it isn't very filling at all. People expecting a filling pasta dish may be left disappointed and still hungry, and who wants that? Also, zucchini requires prep time of salting to remove its bitter juices, otherwise when you cook it, it tends to be both bitter and watery.

Carrots, on the other hand, are a starchy veggie so they're much more filling, and they are usually pretty easy on people's stomachs, especially when cooked. Parsley further aids digestion and lime zest provides both an interesting flavor contrast and some pectin, which also helps you to feel full. Lemon or orange rind would work equally well.

Yield: 2 servings

Ingredients

Scant 1 tablespoon olive oil or ghee
2 cups shredded carrots
1 pinch salt
1 teaspoon chopped parsley
½ teaspoon lime zest

Instructions

1. Heat oil or ghee in a sauté pan over medium-high heat until hot.

2. Add carrots and salt, and toss to coat in fat.

3. Saute until softened and browned, 8 to 10 minutes.

4. Remove from heat and add parsley and lime zest.

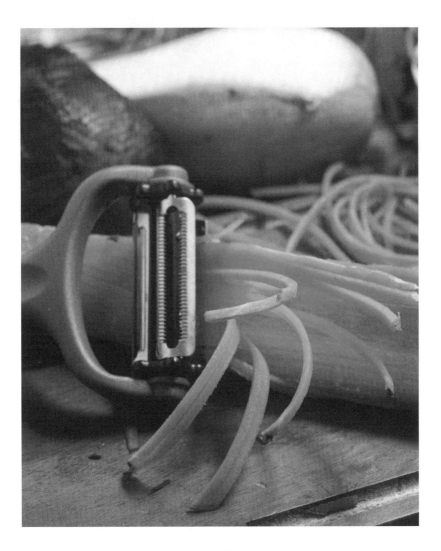

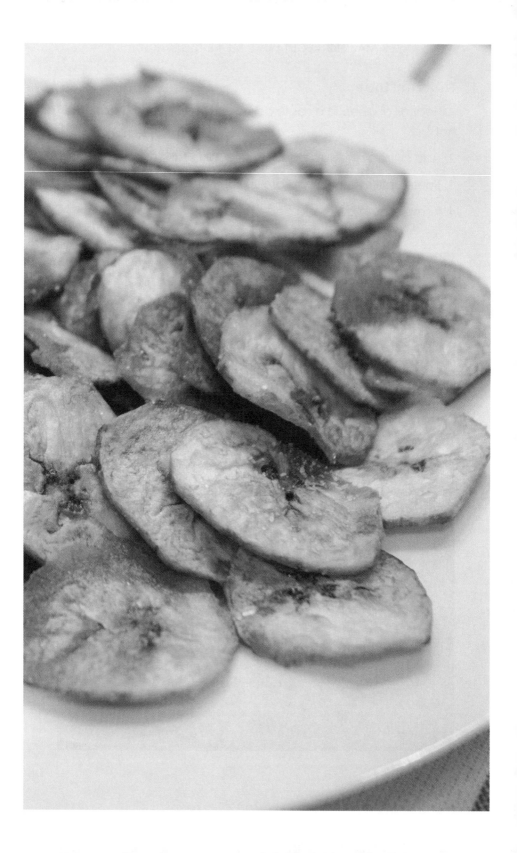

ROASTED PLANTAIN CHIPS

Plantain chips have become a mainstay of the paleo movement, replacing corn or potato chips for those following a "caveman"-style diet that eschews specific tubers and all grains. Unfortunately, when you purchase plantain chips, they're fried just like other store-bought chips. Making them yourself is a quick task, they taste as good as the fried version when you roast them in the oven, and they give you the feeling of eating something indulgent without actually doing so. Compared to corn, plantains offer much more health-wise: They are chock full of fiber and vitamin A, and also don't contribute to inflammation like corn does. These chips are great with anything from guacamole to ceviche, or even on their own for a crunchy snack. You can slice them crosswise or lengthwise, depending on how big a chip you care for.

Yield: 4 servings

Ingredients

2 plantains
1 tablespoon neutral oil, such as avocado or grape seed
½ teaspoon salt

Instructions

1. Preheat oven to 400°F.

2. With a mandoline, food processor, or by hand, slice the plantains into ⅛-inch-thick slices.

3. Drizzle oil on a lined baking sheet, then lay plantain slices onto it. Sprinkle with salt.

4. Roast for 20 minutes, until golden brown.

ROASTED POTATO–STYLE ROOT VEGGIES

This dish is a great choice when you're craving the heaviness and handheld fun of roasted potato wedges but want more health value. There is an array of root vegetables always available in grocery stores, and we don't tend to use them as much as we should, mostly because we don't necessarily know what to do with them. Because they grow in winter, this nourishing vegetable category is usually available no matter where you live.

In addition to the already heralded celery root as a root veggie option here, parsnips have folate and manganese, turnips have lots of fiber and vitamin C, beets have folic acid and magnesium, and rutabagas offer zinc and calcium. Experiment with which you prefer to find the right ones for you. Sweeter choices include parsnips and beets, whereas more savory ones are turnips and rutabagas; it's delicious to combine both flavor elements together, but of course you're free to stick to whichever you prefer.

Yield: 4 servings

Ingredients

4 cups root vegetables, peeled if needed, and cut into ½-inch slices

1 tablespoon neutral oil, such as avocado or grape seed

½ tablespoon Italian herbs

½ teaspoon salt

⅛ teaspoon black pepper

Instructions

1. Preheat oven to 400°F.

2. Lay vegetables out on a lined baking sheet. Drizzle with oil and seasonings.

3. Roast 20 minutes, then remove from oven and stir well.

4. Roast an additional 15 to 20 minutes, until golden and softened.

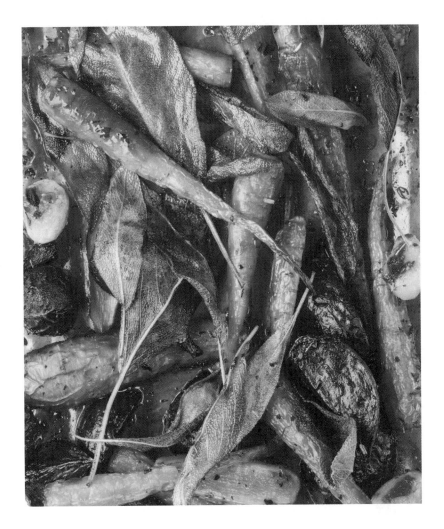

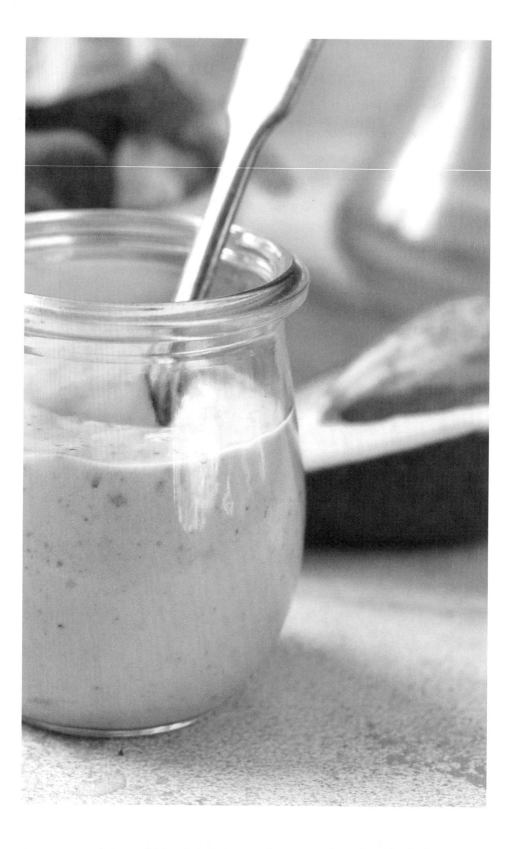

AVOCADO DIGESTIVE DRESSING

When first asked to make this by a client, the idea of blending an avocado with water and some seasonings didn't sound like it could possibly be good. (I've mentioned being an initial tough sell on adding water to food that's perfectly good as is, and this was no exception.) However, I don't always know best, and I'm happy to be proven wrong—and boy was I proven wrong here! This simple dressing is so creamy and delicious, and I actually make it on my own pretty regularly. Lemon juice aids digestion by helping the liver produce bile. Avocado with its fiber and monounsaturated fatty acids is overall wonderful for health, and the avocado's mild taste shines through perfectly here.

Yield: 4 servings

Ingredients

½ cup avocado pulp

¼ cup water (filtered or spring), more if needed

2 tablespoons freshly squeezed lemon juice

¼ teaspoon cumin

1 pinch of salt

⅛ teaspoon black pepper

Instructions

Blend all ingredients in a blender until smooth.

SLOW-COOKED SUNCHOKES

Dubbed "fartichokes" in the culinary world, sunchokes (formerly known as Jerusalem artichokes) are one of the highest foods in beneficial prebiotic fiber. Prebiotic fiber is the food that probiotics eat, meaning that eating these increases the quantity and health of your gut flora without you having to directly consume probiotics. Prebiotics only became a buzz word in the last few years, and many consumers hurried to stock up on prebiotic-rich foods only to discover that suddenly they felt worse than before due to bloating and gas. That's because foods with high prebiotic fiber contents can lead to incredible digestive upset. If you're doing something healthy only to be put in major discomfort, the point is somewhat lost.

The best way to mitigate the potential issues of bloating and gas from prebiotic-rich foods is to break down some of that good fiber, which will still leave plenty behind for you to benefit from, by cooking them slowly. Sunchokes taste like an artichoke and a potato had a baby, and are absolutely heavenly. This recipe lets their deliciousness have its own spot in the sun, but you can add any fresh or dried herbs or spices you love, too.

Yield: 2 servings

Ingredients

3 cups peeled and chopped sunchokes
1 tablespoon neutral oil, such as grape seed or avocado
½ teaspoon salt

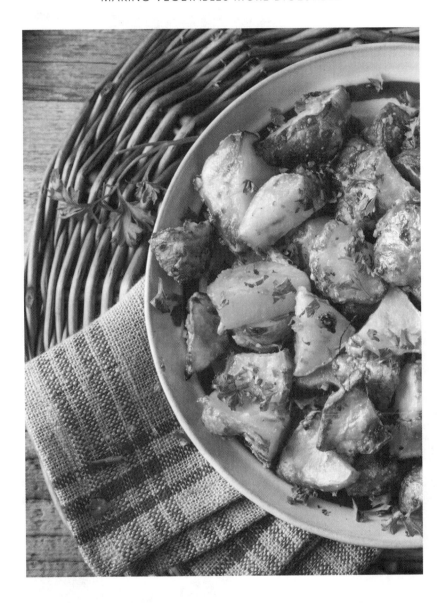

Instructions

1. Preheat oven to 300°F.

2. Place sunchokes on a lined baking sheet and drizzle with oil.

3. Bake for 1½ to 2 hours, until tender and golden.

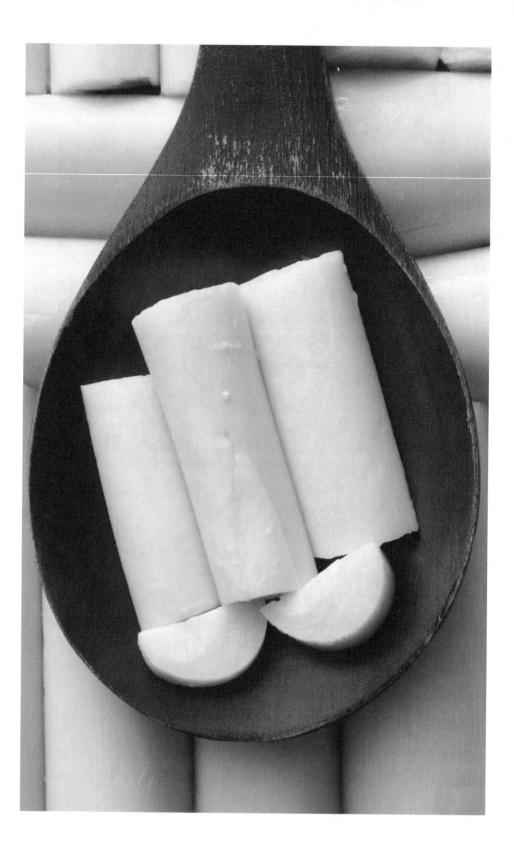

PROBIOTIC HEARTS OF PALM DIP

If you're a fan of artichoke dip, you'll go wild for this incredibly straightforward, less-than-five-minutes-to-make hearts of palm dip. It's thick enough to dip a chip into (I recommend the plantain chips on page 169), and it's surprisingly rich for having so little of a yogurt product in it. The probiotics in yogurt help with digestion of the veggie, which is already easy for your body to assimilate because it's sold cooked (in jars or cans). Low in calories but high in fiber and moderate in protein, hearts of palm also offer manganese and iron in addition to a mild, pleasant flavor. This is another veggie dish that reads as more complex than it is, and it can help satiate a craving for some chips-and-dip–style comfort food without leading to inflammation or digestive upset.

Yield: 4 servings

Ingredients

1 cup hearts of palm
2 tablespoons yogurt (dairy or non)
½ teaspoon garlic powder
¼ teaspoon salt
½ teaspoon black pepper

Instructions

Combine all ingredients in a food processor or blender and pulse until desired texture; mixture should resemble an artichoke dip, mostly creamy with small bits of texture.

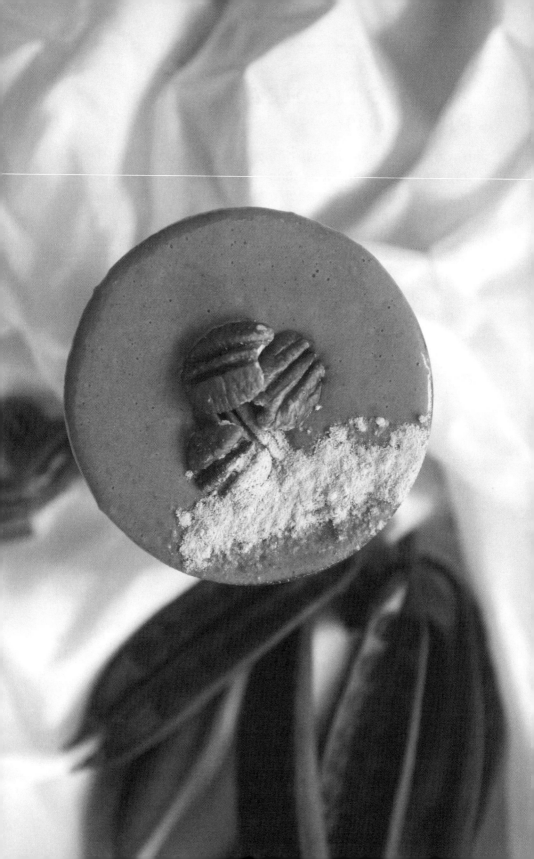

TWELVE
Innocent Desserts

Including a dessert section felt imperative to me for this book because sweet treats are one of the first things to go when our health begins to decline. The standard ingredients in baked goods, such as white wheat flour and cane sugar, are a couple of the biggest contributors to inflammation and gut bacteria imbalance.

You may have already switched out wheat-based treats with gluten-free ones, but unfortunately, those can be equally harmful and hard on your body (unless you are celiac, in which case wheat will surely ruin you). That's because the main ingredients in most commercial gluten-free flour mixes and baked goods are pretty darn unhealthy! They're full of starches and gums, and in much higher concentrations than we have ever consumed such ingredients before in the past. If you think about historic consumption of starch, we'd add something like one teaspoon of corn starch to a stir fry that was large enough to feed a family; now we're buying bagels, cakes, and breads that have corn, arrowroot, tapioca, or potato starch as their preliminary ingredient(s). That means that in a single serving, you're likely eating tablespoons of starch . . . and that's without even factoring in the gums, which are food additives that contribute further to the binding effects of the starches.

Tapioca flour has become the darling of the gluten-free world, but it's a nutrient-void flour (just look on the package) that has a higher glycemic index than sweet potatoes. It is better than tapioca starch, but not by much, and it or its starch counterpart tend to be one of the main ingredients in gluten-free flour mixes and baked goods. It's no surprise that gluten-free baked goods can cause constipation, bloating, and digestive distress.

Here, for the dessert recipes we are going to opt for single, nutrient-rich, whole-food flours. They don't contribute to inflammation, they offer protein and fiber, and while their taste isn't as "white" as either wheat flour or gluten-free starch/gum mixes, all the flours used are mild enough to still make for scrumptious treats while adding to your health rather than taking from it.

Frozen desserts tend to be comprised mostly of either cane sugar or corn syrup, as well as unfermented dairy that can be hard to digest. We'll focus on better ingredients, using noncaloric sweeteners wherever possible and fruit or nuts instead of filler ingredients to bulk up the recipes.

The recipes in this chapter focus more on fruit than anything else, because fruit is a fiber-rich whole food group with a wide range of nutrients. Most fruit is naturally sweet, so little sweetener needs to be added. Because of fruit's fiber content, the sugar is absorbed into your bloodstream more slowly, so you're less likely to experience a blood sugar spike and crash.

These desserts will give you some new options for sweet treats that you can keep on hand without stressing. They store well, so if there is something you particularly enjoy, don't be afraid to batch it up to have on hand for longer.

CHOCO-CADO FUDGE

I didn't plan on this recipe being a winner, let alone on the first try, and neither did my sous chef. "Just avocados and chocolate?" she said, surprised. "That'll really turn into fudge?" I shrugged and hoped for the best, because honestly, throwing some seemingly random stuff together based on an idea I have is my typical creation process. We tasted the first round of this immediately and were super delighted . . . but it was once it had firmed up in the fridge that we got really excited. With so few ingredients, and such healthful ones at that, it really does turn into a fudge.

This recipe can be entirely sugar free if you use stevia-sweetened chocolate chips, unsweetened almond milk, and a noncaloric sweetener, as we did. Chocolate offers a plethora of health benefits, such as antioxidants and balancing the immune system, and contains a small enough amount of caffeine to generally be tolerated even by those who are currently sensitive to coffee (about 12 milligrams per tablespoon of cocoa powder). If you find that chocolate is just not viable for you at all, use carob chips. Avocado has monounsaturated fatty acids that are great for your heart, and grass-fed butter contains butyric acid, a powerful anti-inflammatory agent.

Yield: 10–12 servings

Ingredients

1 cup chocolate chips
1 tablespoon grass-fed butter or coconut oil
½ cup avocado pulp
¼ cup milk (dairy or non—I use almond)
½ teaspoon vanilla extract
Sweetener to taste

Continued . . .

Instructions

1. Melt chocolate chips with butter in a double boiler or over very low heat, stirring frequently.

2. In a blender, combine all remaining ingredients and blend until smooth and creamy.

3. Remove chocolate mixture from heat once completely melted and mix in avocado mixture until uniform in texture and no green or brown lumps remain.

4. Pour fudge into a lined small pan and refrigerate until firm, about 2 hours.

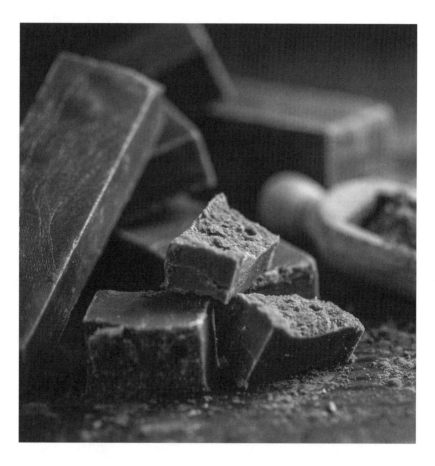

CINNAMON BAKED APPLES

If you're craving apple pie, this dessert is a solid alternative. It couldn't be simpler, and unlike apple pie, there's no reason for any guilt over eating a big serving of it. In fact, you wouldn't even need to feel guilty for having it as breakfast! Apples are one of the highest foods in pectin, which helps lower cholesterol, manage weight, and moderate motility. Coconut sugar has a caramel flavor that pairs perfectly with the apples, while also being considered a slightly healthier alternative to cane sugar. If you're too sensitive for coconut sugar, either omit completely or substitute a noncaloric sweetener such as monk fruit or Swerve.

The water in the baking dish is not imperative, but will help prevent the apples from drying out and can also be used as a sauce for serving. As far as apple choice goes, granny smith are always a safe bet because they are tart and firm; firmness is important so that they keep their shape and don't dissolve into a pile of applesauce. Other good choices include pink lady and braeburn, which also soften without losing shape.

Yield: 2 servings

Ingredients

2 apples, cored
Water sufficient to cover bottom of baking dish
½ tablespoon coconut sugar
1 teaspoon cinnamon

Continued . . .

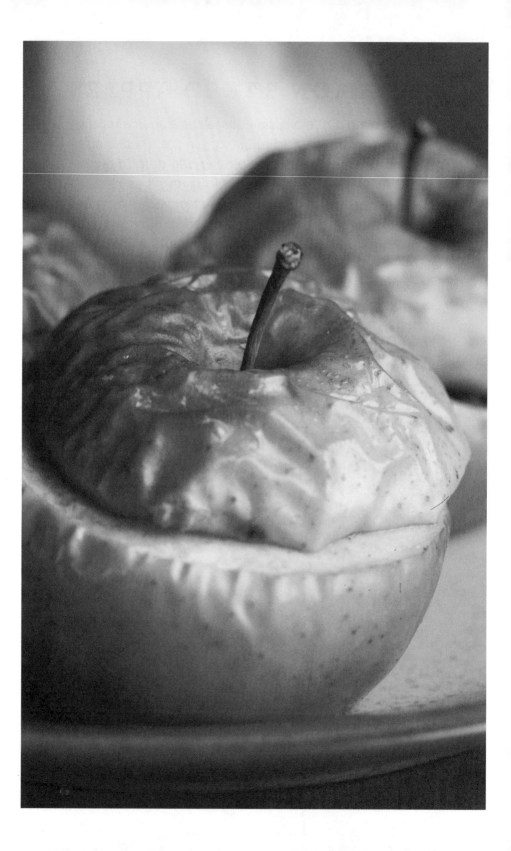

Instructions

1. Preheat oven to 350°F.

2. Place apples in a small baking dish and add enough water to cover the bottom of the dish—barely ⅛ of an inch is plenty.

3. Sprinkle apples with sugar and cinnamon, letting some fall into the cored centers.

4. Bake until wrinkled and soft, about 35 minutes.

COCONUT WHIP PARFAIT

Coconut whipped cream may have peaked in popularity a couple of years ago, but it remains a super-easy way to get the richness and delightfulness of whipped cream without any dairy. You can choose any in-season fruit that agrees with you, or make this particularly good for digestion by opting to include papaya (which has the digestion-affirming enzyme papain). Coconut products are both filling and have a range of benefits a typical whipped cream can't compete with, such as metabolism-boosting, medium-chain triglycerides (discussed on page 122) and anti-fungal properties.

Note that this recipe will only work with canned coconut milk. See pages 108–9 for thoughts on canned foods in Chapter Eight.

Yield: 2 servings

Ingredients

1 can coconut milk, unshaken and refrigerated
Sweetener to taste
½ teaspoon vanilla extract
2 cups chopped fruit of choice

Instructions

1. Place coconut solids in a mixing bowl, discarding liquid underneath.

2. Whip until light and fluffy, about 5 minutes. Alternately, whip with an electric mixer.

3. Add sweetener, such as a few drops of stevia, and vanilla, then combine well.

4. In two bowls or glasses, layer fruit with coconut whipped cream, reserving additional whipped cream for another use.

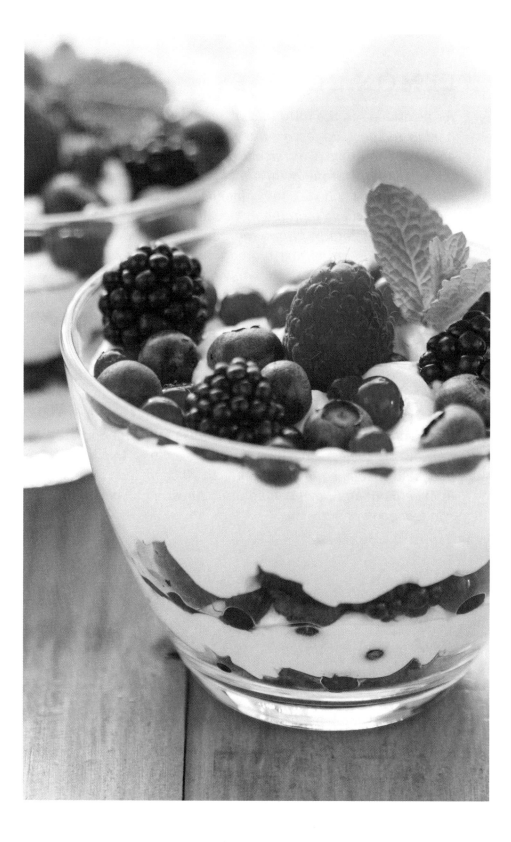

LEMON COOKIES

As mentioned in the intro to this chapter, most gluten-free baking recipes suggest you use a flour mix that contains starches and gums. Conversely, most paleo baking recipes (including most of my own) utilize almond and/or coconut flour. I wanted to offer a simple, inexpensive, but still healthy alternative to these ingredients because some people have issues with tolerating nuts and coconut, so I decided to make a cookie out of just brown rice flour. I was trepidatious because that isn't commonly done, but thankfully my worry was for nothing . . . which is kind of a metaphor for life! The cookie result from just brown rice flour is surprisingly tender, and keeps well; these cookies stayed fresh, fluffy, and wonderfully cakey for nearly a week before drying out, and didn't get moldy in that time at room temperature, either, which almond or coconut flour–based goods usually will. Lemon zest has weight-friendly pectin, and brown rice flour won't contribute to candida or cause inflammation. As I always try to accomplish with dessert recipes, this batter needs no special equipment, and can all be mixed together at once. Fork and bowl baking at its finest, for cookies you can feel good about!

Yield: 9 cookies

Ingredients

1 cup brown rice flour

1 egg

½ cup coconut sugar or Swerve

¼ cup neutral oil, such as avocado or grape seed

½ tablespoon lemon zest

½ teaspoon baking soda

½ teaspoon lemon extract

¼ teaspoon salt

Instructions

1. Preheat oven to 350°F.

2. Mix all ingredients together in a mixing bowl until uniform in texture.

3. Dollop onto a lined baking sheet, dividing into nine cookies.

4. Bake until firm and golden, about 12 minutes.

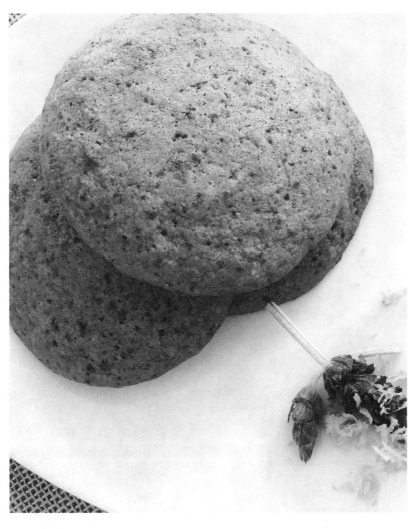

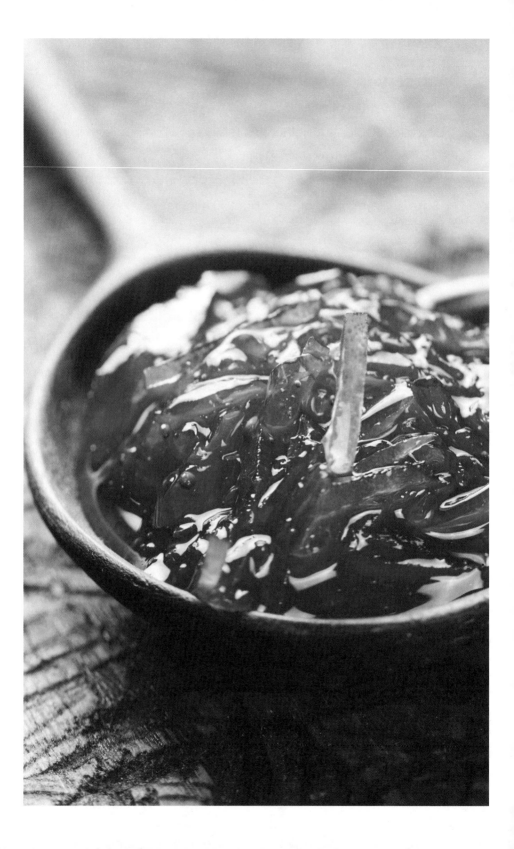

SPICED ORANGE SAUCE

While it's important to have dessert recipes that are just plain yummy, I also wanted to make sure to include ones with function. I love small bites of something sweet at the end of a meal, especially when I'm too full for dessert but still want to end on a refreshing note. Orange peel is used regularly as a digestive aid, so there is a lot of it hidden in this sauce. The recipe can be eaten alone as a post-meal sweet bite, or used as a topping for another dessert such as cake or ice cream. Think orange marmalade, only a lot brighter in flavor. Cinnamon will help stabilize blood sugar, so you don't experience too much of a spike and drop of it after having eaten, and cardamom gives the dish an exotic edge while counteracting bloating and heartburn. For added antibacterial benefit, choose manuka honey over regular if possible for you from a budget standpoint.

Yield: 2 servings

Ingredients

¾ cup orange segments (about 1 medium orange), cut into
   thirds
2 tablespoons orange zest
1 tablespoon freshly squeezed orange juice
1 teaspoon manuka or regular honey
¼ teaspoon cinnamon
⅛ teaspoon cardamom

Instructions

Mix all ingredients together and let marinate for at least
10 minutes.

PECAN PIE MILKSHAKE

When I came up with the idea for this recipe, I scoured the Internet for versions both healthy and junk food-y, as I often do to see what people are loving. When I saw the ingredients in a "normal" pecan pie milkshake—including ice cream, pieces of actual pecan pie, and often even a shot of bourbon—my confidence sank. How could I make a whole-food version that would compare? It took a couple of tries, but I'm happy to say, this healthy milkshake makes for SUCH a solid dessert! Full of protein and the beneficial spices that make up pumpkin pie spice mix, and without the need for additional sweetener thanks to what's not even that large a quantity of bananas and dates, you can re-create a holiday indulgence anytime. Because this smoothie has energizing carbs plus plenty of protein, it beats the pants off a doughnut or muffin as an indulgent breakfast treat!

Yield: 2 servings

Ingredients

¾ cup milk (dairy or non)

2 dates

3 teaspoons roasted pecans

¼ cup frozen banana pieces

3 ice cubes

½ teaspoon pumpkin pie spice

2 scoops vanilla protein powder

1 small pinch salt

½ teaspoon maple syrup, optional

Instructions

Blend all ingredients in a blender until smooth and creamy.

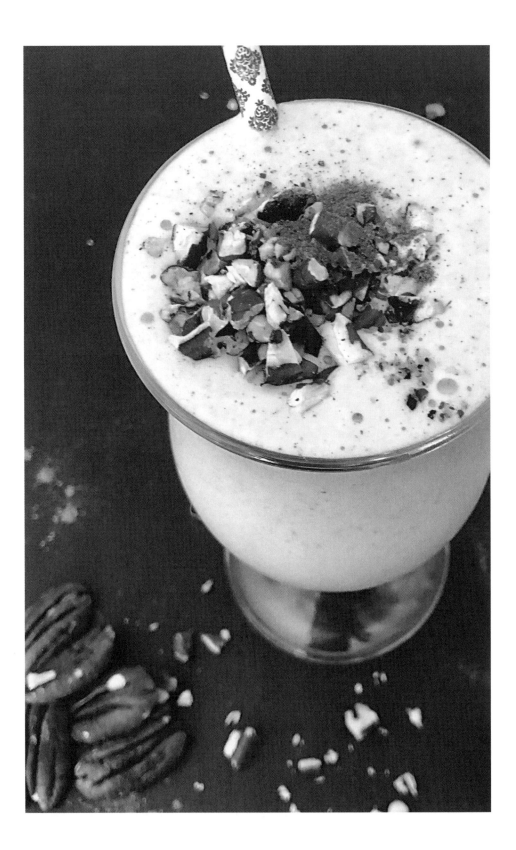

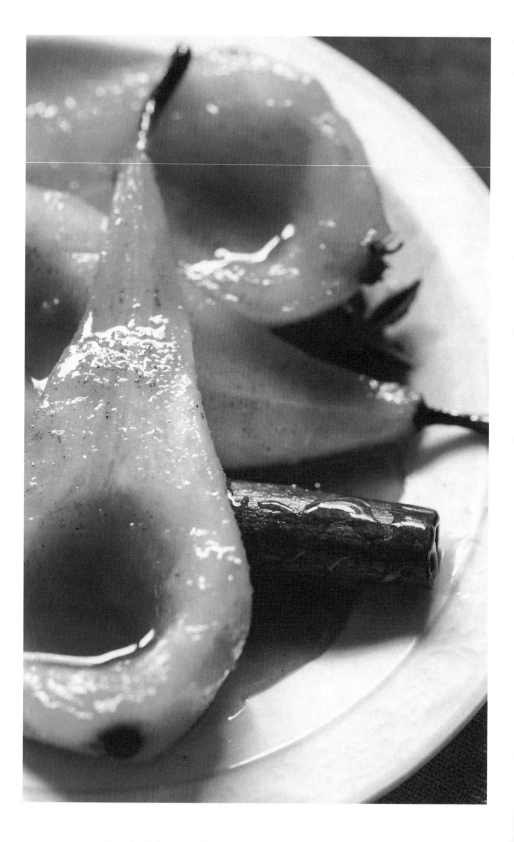

BRAISED PEARS

As simple as baked apples, this dish has more of an elegant appearance than a homey one. The braising process makes a heavenly aroma as the pears cook—feel free to add some hard spices such as cardamom pods or a couple of cloves for a take that's holiday appropriate, yet far lighter and healthier than a normal holiday dessert would be. As a high-fiber fruit, pears are a good choice for those who find they have a glycemic response (sugar high then crash) from dessert items. They're great for inflammation, as well as for relieving constipation.

I like to serve this on a plate, sliced so you can see the color difference between inside and outside. Even if you don't use tea or berries for color, the outsides still darken from cooking. Adding a heaping spoonful of the Spiced Orange Sauce (page 191) will contribute further to this being a "fancy" dessert that's as good for you as a fruit cup.

Yield: 4 servings

Ingredients

2 pears, peeled, cored, and sliced in half lengthwise

½ cup freshly squeezed orange juice

2 tablespoons freshly squeezed lemon juice

½ cup water, or more if needed

2 tablespoons honey or maple syrup

Optional for color: 1 serving hibiscus tea or a handful of berries

Instructions

1. In a saucepot over medium-high heat, add all ingredients and bring to a boil.

2. Reduce to a simmer, remove tea or berries if using, and simmer until pears have softened slightly, about 10 minutes.

MELON POPS

Popsicles are a treat that most find nostalgic. No matter what your upbringing was, chances are you occasionally had a frozen fruit treat you could hold in your hands. In the summer months, popsicles quenched our thirst, offered us hydration, were fun to consume, and tasted like heaven. This version is quick to make, doesn't require any additional sweetener because melons are inherently so sweet, and stores well in the freezer if kept in the molds. You'll most likely find that they don't have an opportunity to hang around for long, though! I love making a big batch of them with multiple types of melons, which you can do either alone or layered into the molds. Watermelon will have the iciest result, and is notable for its lycopene content, which aids in everything from diabetes to heart issues, because it is particularly easy for your body to absorb over other produce items that contain it. More fleshy melons such as cantaloupe or honeydew will give you a creamier popsicle. If you got excited enough to buy a big melon in season, then came home and got concerned about eating it all, this is the perfect use for some of it.

Note: *Melon seeds can be eaten and are totally healthful! If you're feeling adventurous, save the seeds from your melon and roast them. This is the only step needed for cantaloupe, honeydew, or other melon with soft seeds. If choosing watermelon, the outer shell needs to be removed first, which can be done by boiling them first for a few minutes, then cooling and peeling them. You can then roast them as you would other melon seeds. They contain multiple antioxidants, and in good concentration.*

Yield: 6 servings

Ingredients

2 cups chopped melon

½ cup filtered or spring water

Lemon juice or sweetener to taste

Instructions

1. Blend all ingredients until smooth.

2. Pour into popsicle molds and freeze until firm, 4 to 6 hours.

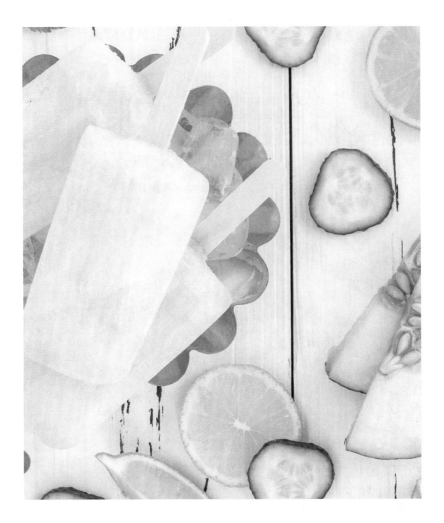

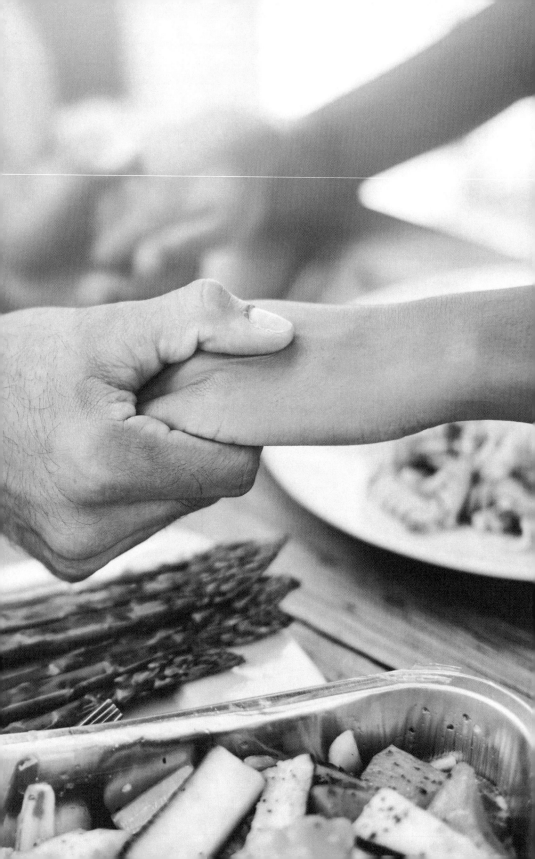

Conclusion

My, what an experience this has been! I don't know the last time I've gone through such a wringer of emotions in one writing piece, but my overwhelming emotion right now is one of hope: I'm full of hope that by having read this book, you feel as exhilarated and excited about your wellness as I do for you.

You may be feeling a little overwhelmed, which is normal; my goal whenever I talk about wellness with people is to offer them as many options and tools as possible. I do that because naturally, some are bound to stick out more than others, and I think that you should begin with whichever tool is most in the forefront of your brain, ready for you, that you're thinking about with the most enthusiasm. Do what excites you most; it will yield the best results.

Ideally, you'll do as many exercises in this book as it takes for you to get onto a solid track for recovery, and you'll keep doing them until you feel like a million bucks (which by now you may actually believe is possible!). That may be one per chapter's worth, or it may be all. You might make one recipe, love it, and have it daily for years, or you might try a couple dozen then move on to someone else's healing recipes. There is no right or wrong answer for how to use this book; it exists for you, and I wrote it to be used however will best serve you. I intentionally avoid strict protocols in my work because I want your path to wellness to be about you empowering you, not me instructing you.

It's my biggest desire and ultimate goal that *How to Be Well When You're Not* has brought you, at the very least, some relief in the knowledge that you are not alone. Whatever you're experiencing, you are not alone in it, even if you can't see anyone else around right now going through it. Somewhere in the world, they picked up this book too! No matter how unwell you're feeling, please don't forget that we are all just humans, doing the best we can with our own little lives, striving to be our best, and longing to connect with something greater than ourselves.

You are good enough. You deserve to be in perfect health. Whether you see yourself as full of shortcomings, or made of pure magic, I believe we are all the latter no matter how many we have of the former. If nothing else, I hope this book has helped you to spend time learning how to believe in yourself. No one has more power to help you be well than you do; if this book has made your wellness seem more viable—and of course my goal is that it has, in as many ways as possible—that's just me acting as a conduit for the skills and knowledge that already exist deep within your cells. Someday, you could be documenting your wellness story, helping others to find their paths to health. There is no limit to what any of us can accomplish.

May you be well, even when you're not.

All my love,
Ariane

Acknowledgments

While there are countless people who have loved me into being the person capable of writing this book, there are a select few who made the reality of it possible.

My literary agent Coleen O'Shea: This is our third book together, and has me confident in that old "Three's a charm" saying. Thank you for your continued support.

Ann Treistman at The Countryman Press: Thank you for leading the conversation right into this book; it existing is my dream come true.

Róisín Cameron, my editor at The Countryman Press: Thank you for never making me feel like my kids are being killed off.

Alecia/P!nk: I regularly thank the two whiskey drinks that gave me the courage to ask you about writing the foreword to this book, and I thank you for all you've taught me even more often.

Mandy: You're my favorite sous chef ever, and real high on my favorite-people-ever list.

Philipe: The ways I've grown by working with you have facilitated my writing in innumerable ways.

My family: You are where my purpose was found, and your pride fuels me.

Sat Devbir Singh: My magical star seed sibling, I don't even want to think about where I'd be without you.

My people: There's a good bunch of you between SF and LA and NYC, and I know you'll see this; you always buy my books because you are wonderful friends. Thank you for your unwavering presence in my life.

Chanty and Bechamel: Without you I'd just be a crazy cat-less lady. Thank you for all the cuddles as I slogged through the hard parts of writing.

Most of all: You, dear reader. Without you, I'd just be a girl having a really long conversation with herself. Thank you for giving my life purpose.

Resources

Introduction

Goodin, B. R., T. Kronfli, C. D. King, T. L. Glover, K. Sibille, and R. B. Fillingim. "Testing the relation between dispositional optimism and conditioned pain modulation: does ethnicity matter?" *Journal of Behavioral Medicine*, 2013, 36(2): link.springer.com/article/10.1007%2Fs10865-012-9411-7.

Levy, B. R. and A. Bavishi. "Survival Advantage Mechanism: Inflammation as a Mediator of Positive Self-Perceptions of Aging on Longevity." *The Journals of Gerontology: Series B*, 2018, 73(3): academic.oup.com/psych-socgerontology/article-abstract/73/3/409/2631978.

Mondloch, M. V., D. C. Cole, and J. W. Frank. "Does how you do depend on how you think you'll do? A systematic review of the evidence for a relation between patients' recovery expectations and health outcomes." *Canadian Medical Association Journal*, 2001, 165(2): 174–79.

Young, P. H. Yuchi, Barbara Resnick, PhD, Rehabil Nurs. "Don't Worry and Be Positive: What helps the most in functional recovery one year after hip fracture? An exit interview." *PMC*, 2009, 34(3): www.ncbi.nlm.nih.gov/pmc/articles/PMC2729270/.

Chapter Six

Ekeocha, T. C. "The Effects of Visualization and Guided Imagery in Sports Performance." Graduate Council of Texas State University, May 2015: digital.library.txstate.edu/bitstream/handle/10877/5548/EKEOCHA-THESIS-2015.pdf?sequence=1.

Karns C. M, W. E. Moore III, U. Mayr. "The Cultivation of Pure Altruism via Gratitude: A Functional MRI Study of Change with Gratitude Practice." *Front Hum Neurosci*, 2017 Dec 12: www.ncbi.nlm.nih.gov/pubmed/29375336.

Petrocchi, N. and A. Couyoumdjian. "The impact of gratitude on depression and anxiety: the mediating role of criticizing, attacking, and reassuring the self." *Self and Identity*, 2016, 15(2): www.tandfonline.com/doi/full/10.1080/15298868.2015.1095794.

Ranganathan V. K., V. Siemionow, J. Z. Liu, V. Sahgal, G. H. Yue. "From mental power to muscle power–gaining strength by using the mind." *Neuropsychologia*, 2004: www.ncbi.nlm.nih.gov/pubmed/14998709.

Redwine L. S., Henry B. L., Pung M. A., Wilson K., Chinh K., Knight B., Jain S., Rutledge T., Greenberg B., Maisel A., Mills P. J. "Pilot Randomized Study of a Gratitude Journaling Intervention on Heart Rate Variability and Inflammatory Biomarkers in Patients with Stage B Heart Failure." *Psychosom Med*, 2016 Jul–Aug: www.ncbi.nlm.nih.gov/pubmed/27187845.

Chapter Seven

Behringer, M., D. Jedlicka, M. McCourt, M. Ring, and J. Mester. "Effects of lymphatic drainage and local cryo exposition regeneration after high-intensive exercises." *Muscles Ligaments Tendons Journal*, 2016 Apr–Jun: www.ncbi.nlm.nih.gov/pmc/articles/PMC5115255/.

Booth, F. W., C. K. Roberts, and M. J. Laye. "Lack of exercise is a major cause of chronic diseases." *Compr Physiol*, 2012 Apr: www.ncbi.nlm.nih.gov/pmc/articles/PMC4241367/.

Chase N. L., X. Sui, and S. N. Blair. "Swimming and all-cause mortality risk compared with running, walking, and sedentary habits in men." *International Journal of Aquatic Research and Education*, 2008, 2(3): scholarworks.bgsu.edu/cgi/viewcontent.cgi?referer=https://www.google.com/&httpsredir=1&article=1247&context=ijare.

Church, D. "Emotional Freedom Techniques to Treat Post-traumatic Stress Disorder in Veterans: Review of the Evidence, Survey of Practitioners, and Proposed Clinical Guidelines." *The Permanente Journal*, 2017: www.ncbi.nlm.nih.gov/pmc/articles/PMC5499602/.

Cider A., B. G. Svealv, M. S. Tang, M. Schaufelberger, and B. Andersson. "Immersion in warm water induces improvement in cardiac function in patients with chronic heart failure." *Eur J Heart Fail*, 2006 May: www.ncbi.nlm.nih.gov/pubmed/16256434.

Giampietro L. V., S. J. Miller, N. M. McBrier, and W. E. Buckley. "Systematic Review of Efficacy for Manual Lymphatic Drainage Techniques in Sports Medicine and Rehabilitation: An Evidence-Based Practice Approach." *J Man Manip Ther*, 2009: www.ncbi.nlm.nih.gov/pmc/articles/PMC2755111/.

Hall J., S. M. Skevington, P. J. Maddison, and K. Chapman. "A randomized and controlled trial of hydrotherapy in rheumatoid arthritis." *Arthritis Care Res*, 1996–1999: www.ncbi.nlm.nih.gov/pubmed/8971230.

Harber, V. J. and J. R. Sutton. "Endorphins and exercise." *Sports Med*, 1984 Mar–Apr: www.ncbi.nlm.nih.gov/pubmed/6091217.

Herrero, J. L., S. Khuvis, E. Yeagle, M. Cerf, and A. D. Mehta. "Breathing above the brain stem: volitional control and attentional modulation in humans." *Journal of Neurophysiology*, 3 Jan 2018: www.physiology.org/doi/abs/10.1152/jn.00551.2017.

Jerath R., J. W. Edry, V. A. Barnes, V. Jerath. "Physiology of long pranayamic breathing: neural respiratory elements may provide a mechanism that explains how slow deep breathing shifts the autonomic nervous system." *Med Hypotheses*, 2006 April: www.ncbi.nlm.nih.gov/pubmed/16624497.

Kim, Y.-D., I. Heo, B.-C. Shin, C. Crawford, H.-W. Kang, and J.-H. Lim. "Acupuncture for Post-traumatic Stress Disorder: A Systematic Review of Randomized Controlled Trials and Prospective Clinical Trials." *Evid Based Complement Alternat Med*, 2013: www.ncbi.nlm.nih.gov/pmc/articles/PMC3580897/.

Knab A. M., R. A. Shanely, K. D. Corbin, F. Jin, W. Sha, D. C. Nieman. "A 45-minute vigorous exercise bout increases metabolic rate for 14 hours." *Med Sci Sports Exerc*, 2011 Sep: www.ncbi.nlm.nih.gov/pubmed/21311363.

Köroğlu, M. and K. Yiğiter. "Effects of Swimming Training on Stress Levels of the Students Aged 11-13" *Universal Journal of Educational Research*, 2016: files.eric.ed.gov/fulltext/EJ1110780.pdf.

Kox M., M. Stoffels, S. P. Smeekens, N. van Alfen, M. Gomes, T. M. Eijsvogels, M. T. Hopman, J. G. van der Hoeven, M. G. Netea, P. Pickkers. "The influence of concentration/meditation on autonomic nervous system activity and the innate immune response: a case study." *Psychosom Med*, 2012 Jun: www.ncbi.nlm.nih.gov/pubmed/22685240.

Lane, K., D. Worsley, and D. McKenzie. "Exercise and the Lymphatic System Implications for Breast-Cancer Survivors." *Sports Med*, 2005: pdfs.semanticscholar.org/b639/33b46c2652aea354006704ad504a361b9d39.pdf.

Puetz, T. W., P. J. O'Connor, R. K. Dishman. "Effects of chronic exercise on feelings of energy and fatigue: A quantitative synthesis." *Psychological Bulletin*, 2006, 132(6): psycnet.apa.org/buy/2006-20202-002.

Roman G., M. Quintana, M. Engardt, L. Gullstrand, E. Jansson, and L. Kaijser. "Older women's cardiovascular responses to deep-water running." *Aging Phys Act*, 2006: www.ncbi.nlm.nih.gov/pubmed/16648650.

Sanders, R. "If you 'feel the burn,' you need to bulk up your mitochondria." Media Relations: UC Berekley Press Release, 19 April 2006: www.berkeley.edu/news/media/releases/2006/04/19_lactate.shtml.

Vickers, A. J., A. M. Cronin, A. C. Maschino. "Acupuncture for Chronic Pain Individual Patient Data Meta-analysis." *Arch Intern Med*, 2012: jamanetwork.com/journals/jamainternalmedicine/fullarticle/1357513.

Chapter Nine

Ayrle, H., M. Mevissen, M. Kaske, H. Nathues, N. Gruetzner, M. Melzig, and M. Walkenhorst. "Medicinal plants–prophylactic and therapeutic options for gastrointestinal and respiratory diseases in calves and piglets? A systematic review." *BMC Vet Res*, 2016: www.ncbi.nlm.nih.gov/pmc/articles/PMC4896019/.

Cai H., X. Chen, J. Zhang, J. Wang. "18β-glycyrrhetinic acid inhibits migration and invasion of human gastric cancer cells via the ROS/PKC-α/ERK pathway." *J Nat Med*, 2018 Jan: www.ncbi.nlm.nih.gov/pubmed/29098529.

Chainani-Wu, N. "Safety and anti-inflammatory activity of curcumin: a component of turmeric (Curcuma longa)." *J Altern Complement Med*, 2003 Feb: www.ncbi.nlm.nih.gov/pubmed/12676044.

Dugasani S., M. R. Pichika, V. D. Nadarajah, M. K. Balijepalli, S. Tandra, and J. N. Korlakunta. "Comparative antioxidant and anti-inflammatory effects of [6]-gingerol, [8]-gingerol, [10]-gingerol and [6]-shogaol." *J Ethnopharmacol*, 2010 Feb 3: www.ncbi.nlm.nih.gov/pubmed/19833188.

Henrotin, Y., F. Priem, and A. Mobasheri. "Curcumin: a new paradigm and therapeutic opportunity for the treatment of osteoarthritis: curcumin for osteoarthritis management." *Springerplus*, 2013: www.ncbi.nlm.nih.gov/pmc/articles/PMC3591524/.

Jamshidi, N., and M. M. Cohen. "The Clinical Efficacy and Safety of Tulsi in Humans: A Systematic Review of the Literature." *Evid Based Complement Alternat Med*, 2017: www.ncbi.nlm.nih.gov/pmc/articles/PMC5376420/.

Jurenka J. S. "Anti-inflammatory properties of curcumin, a major constituent of Curcuma longa: a review of preclinical and clinical research." *Altern Med Rev*, 2009 Jun: www.ncbi.nlm.nih.gov/pubmed/19594223.

Kemmerich, B., R. Eberhardt, H. Stammer. "Efficacy and tolerability of a fluid extract combination of thyme herb and ivy leaves and matched placebo in adults suffering from acute bronchitis with productive cough. A prospective, double-blind, placebo-controlled clinical trial." *Arzneimittelforschung*, 2006; 56(9): 652–60.

Lee, H. H., S. Lee, K. Lee, Y. S. Shin, H. Kang, and H. Cho. "Anti-cancer effect of Cordyceps militaris in human colorectal carcinoma RKO cells via cell cycle arrest and mitochondrial apoptosis." *Daru*, 2015: www.ncbi.nlm.nih.gov/pmc/articles/PMC4491205/.

Lete, I., and J. Allué. "The Effectiveness of Ginger in the Prevention of Nausea and Vomiting during Pregnancy and Chemotherapy." *Integr Med Insights*, 2016: www.ncbi.nlm.nih.gov/pmc/articles/PMC4818021/.

Medagama, A. B. "The glycaemic outcomes of Cinnamon, a review of the experimental evidence and clinical trials." *Nutrition Journal*, 2015: www.ncbi.nlm.nih.gov/pmc/articles/PMC4609100/.

Mohd S. A. K., I. Ahmad, S. S. Cameotra, and F. Botha. "Sub-MICs of Carum copticum and Thymus vulgaris influence virulence factors and biofilm formation in Candida spp." *BMC Complement Altern Med*, 2014: www.ncbi.nlm.nih.gov/pmc/articles/PMC4177179/.

Nagata J. I., C. Kuroiwa, S. Tamaru-Hase, K. Koba. "Effects of Medium Chain Triacylglycerols on the Pathological Condition and Energy Bioavailability of Streptozotocin-induced Diabetic Rats." *J Oleo Sci*, 2018: www.ncbi.nlm.nih.gov/pubmed/29607889.

Ohta Y., N. Kawate, T. Inaba , H. Morii, K. Takahashi, and H. Tamada. "Feeding hydroalcoholic extract powder of Lepidium meyenii (maca) enhances testicular gene expression of 3β-hydroxysteroid dehydrogenase in rats." *Andrologia*, 2017 Dec: www.ncbi.nlm.nih.gov/pubmed/28261840.

Patton T., J. Barrett, J. Brennan, and N. Moran. "Use of a spectrophotometric bioassay for determination of microbial sensitivity to manuka honey." *J Microbiol Methods*, 2006: www.ncbi.nlm.nih.gov/pubmed /15979745.

Rahman, M. A., N. Abdullah, and N. Aminudin. "Inhibitory Effect on In Vitro LDL Oxidation and HMG Co-A Reductase Activity of the Liquid-Liquid Partitioned Fractions of Hericium erinaceus (Bull.) Persoon (Lion's Mane Mushroom)." *Biomed Res Int*, 2014: www.ncbi.nlm.nih.gov/pmc/articles/PMC4052699/.

Sherry C. J., L. E. Ray, R. E. Herron. "The pharmacological effects of the ligroin extract of nutmeg (Myristica fragrans)." *J Ethnopharmacol*, 1982 Jul: www.ncbi.nlm.nih.gov/pubmed/7202086.

Tomljenovic, L. "Aluminum and Alzheimer's disease: after a century of controversy, is there a plausible link?" *J Alzheimers Dis*, 2011, 23(4): 567–98.

Zhanga, L., and B. L. Lokeshwar. "Medicinal Properties of the Jamaican Pepper Plant Pimenta dioica and Allspice." *Curr Drug Targets*. Author manuscript; available in *PMC*, 2014 Jan 14: www.ncbi.nlm.nih.gov/pmc/articles/PMC3891794/.

Živkovič L., V. Bajić, D. Dekanski, A. Čabarkapa-Pirković, F. Giampieri, M. Gasparrini, L. Mazzoni, and B. S. Potparević. "Manuka honey attenuates oxidative damage induced by H2O2 in human whole blood in vitro." *Food Chem Toxicol*, 2018 Sep: www.ncbi.nlm.nih.gov/pubmed/29763681.

Chapter Ten

Clifford, T., C. M. Constantinou, K. M. Keane, D. J. West, G. Howatson, and E. J. Stevenson. "The plasma bioavailability of nitrate and betanin from Beta vulgaris rubra in humans." *Eur J Nutr*, 2017: www.ncbi.nlm.nih.gov/pmc/articles/PMC5346430/.

Clifford, T., G. Howatson, D. J. West, and E. J. Stevenson. "The Potential Benefits of Red Beetroot Supplementation in Health and Disease." *Nutrients*, 2015 Apr: www.ncbi.nlm.nih.gov/pmc/articles/PMC4425174/.

Gao. C. H., J. Q. Qu, X. Y. Zhou, and T. S. Gao. "Iodine-Rich Herbs and Potassium Iodate Have Different Effects on the Oxidative Stress and Differentiation of TH17 Cells in Iodine-Deficient NOD.H-2h Mice." *Biol Trace Elem Res*, 2018 May: www.ncbi.nlm.nih.gov/pubmed/28803408.

Ishigurokuro, K., R. Kurata, Y. Shimada, Y. Sameshima, and T. Kume. "Effects of a sweet potato protein digeston lipid metabolism in mice administered a high-fat diet." *Heliyon*, 2016 2(12): dx.doi.org/10.1016/j.heliyon.2016.e00201.

Larijani, B., M. M. Esfahani, M. Moghimi, M. R. S. Ardakani, M. Keshavarz, G. Kordafshari, E. Nazem, S. H. Ranjbar, H. M. Kenari, and A. Zargaran. "Prevention and Treatment of Flatulence From a Traditional Persian Medicine Perspective." *Iran Red Crescent Med J*, 2016 Apr: www.ncbi.nlm.nih.gov/pmc/articles/PMC4893422/.

Li, C. C., H. F. Yu, C. H. Chang, Y. T. Liu, H. T. Yao. "Effects of lemongrass oil and citral on hepatic drug-metabolizing enzymes, oxidative stress, and acetaminophen toxicity in rats." *J Food Drug Anal*, 2018 Jan: www.ncbi.nlm.nih.gov/pubmed/29389585.

Lima, E. B. C., C. N. S. Sousa, L. N. Meneses, N. C. Ximenes, M. A. Santos, G. S. Vasconcelos, N. B. C. Lima, M. C. A. Patrocínio, D. Macedo, and S. M. M. Vasconcelos. "Cocos nucifera (L.) (Arecaceae): A phytochemical and pharmacological review." *Braz J Med Biol Res*, 2015 Nov: www .ncbi.nlm.nih.gov/pmc/articles/PMC4671521/.

Park, K. H., J. R. Kim, J. S. Lee, H. Lee, and K. H. Cho. "Ethanol and water extract of purple sweet potato exhibits anti-atherosclerotic activity and inhibits protein glycation." *J Med Food*, 2010 Feb: www.ncbi.nlm.nih.gov/ pubmed/20136441.

Scaldaferri, F., L. R. Lopetuso, V. Petito, V. Cufino, M. Bilotta, V. Arena, E. Stigliano, G. Maulucci, M. Papi, C. M. Emiliana, A. Poscia, F. Franceschi, G. Delogu, M. Sanguinetti, M. de Spirito, A. Sgambato, and A. Gasbarrini. "Gelatin tannate ameliorates acute colitis in mice by reinforcing mucus layer and modulating gut microbiota composition: Emerging role for 'gut barrier protectors' in IBD?" *United European Gastroenterol J*, 2014 Apr: www.ncbi.nlm.nih.gov/pmc/articles/PMC4040816/.

Shah, G., R. Shri, V. Panchal, N. Sharma, B. Singh, and A. S. Mann. "Scientific basis for the therapeutic use of Cymbopogon citratus, stapf (Lemon grass)." *J Adv Pharm Technol Res*, 2011 Jan–Mar: www.ncbi.nlm.nih.gov/ pmc/articles/PMC3217679/.

Chapter Eleven

Cherng, S. C., Y. H. Chen, M. S. Lee, S. P. Yang, W. S. Huang, and C. Y. Cheng. "Acceleration of hepatobiliary excretion by lemon juice on 99mTc-tetrofosmin cardiac SPECT." *Nucl Med Commun*, 2006 Nov: www.ncbi .nlm.nih.gov/pubmed/17021425.

Kreydiyyeh, S. I., and J. Usta. "Diuretic effect and mechanism of action of parsley." *J Ethnopharmacol*, 2002 Mar: www.ncbi.nlm.nih.gov/ pubmed/11849841.

Kreydiyyeh, S. I., J. Usta, I. Kaouk, and R. Al-Sadi. "The mechanism underlying the laxative properties of parsley extract." *Phytomedicine*, 2001 Sep: www.ncbi.nlm.nih.gov/pubmed/11695882.

Morsy, T. A., A. E. Kholif, O. H. Matloup, A. Abu Elella, U. Y. Anele, J. S. Caton. "Mustard and cumin seeds improve feed utilisation, milk production and milk fatty acids of Damascus goats." *J Dairy Res*, 2018 May: www.ncbi .nlm.nih.gov/pubmed/29478424.

Wanders, A. J., M. Mars, K. J. Borgonjen-van den Berg, C. de Graaf, and E. J. Feskens. "Satiety and energy intake after single and repeated exposure to gel-forming dietary fiber: post-ingestive effects." *Int J Obes*, 2014 Jun: www.ncbi.nlm.nih.gov/pubmed/24030518.

Chapter Twelve

Abdullah, M. M. H., S. Jew, and P. J. H. Jones. "Health benefits and evaluation of healthcare cost savings if oils rich in monounsaturated fatty acids were substituted for conventional dietary oils in the United States." *Nutr Rev*, 2017 Mar: www.ncbi.nlm.nih.gov/pmc/articles/PMC5914363/.

Borycka-Kiciak, K., T. Banasiewicz, and G. Rydzewska. "Butyric acid—a well-known molecule revisited." *Prz Gastroenterol*, 2017: www.ncbi.nlm.nih.gov/pmc/articles/PMC5497138/.

Camps-Bossacoma, M., F. J. Pérez-Cano, À. Franch, and M. Castell. "Theobromine Is Responsible for the Effects of Cocoa on the Antibody Immune Status of Rats." *J Nutr*, 2018 Mar: www.ncbi.nlm.nih.gov/pubmed/29546302.

Jamal A., K. Javed, M. Aslam, and M. A. Jafri. "Gastroprotective effect of cardamom, Elettaria cardamomum Maton. fruits in rats." *J Ethnopharmacol*, 2006 Jan: www.ncbi.nlm.nih.gov/pubmed/16298093.

Jiang, T., X. Gao, C. Wu, F. Tian, Q. Lei, J. Bi, Bi. Xie, H. Y. Wang, S. Chen, and X. Wang. "Apple-Derived Pectin Modulates Gut Microbiota, Improves Gut Barrier Function, and Attenuates Metabolic Endotoxemia in Rats with Diet-Induced Obesity." *Nutrients*, 2016 Mar: www.ncbi.nlm.nih.gov/pmc/articles/PMC4808856/.

Naz, A., M. S. Butt, M. T. Sultan, M. M. N. Qayyum, and R. S. Niaz. "Watermelon lycopene and allied health claims." *EXCLI J*, 2014: www.ncbi.nlm.nih.gov/pmc/articles/PMC4464475/.

Reiland, H., and J. Slavin. "Systematic Review of Pears and Health." *Nutr Today*, 2015 Nov: ww.ncbi.nlm.nih.gov/pmc/articles/PMC4657810/.

Resnick, A. "What Is Cassava Flour and Why You Should Avoid It." Livestrong.com, 2016 Mar: https://www.livestrong.com/article/1011824-cassava-flour-should-avoid/.

Silva, A. G., R. C.Wanderley, A. F.Pedroso, and G. Ashbell. "Ruminal digestion kinetics of citrus peel." *Animal Feed Science and Technology*, 1997, 68(3–4): www.sciencedirect.com/science/article/pii/S0377840197000564.

Thebo, N. K., A. A. Simair, G. S. Mangrio, K. A. Ansari, A. A. Bhutto, C. Lu, and W. A. Sheikh. "Antifungal Potential and Antioxidant Efficacy in the Shell Extract of Cocos nucifera L. (Arecaceae) against Pathogenic Dermal Mycosis." *Medicines* (Basel), 2016 Jun: www.ncbi.nlm.nih.gov/pmc/articles/PMC5456225/.

Toro-Uribe. S., L. J. López-Giraldo, E. A. Decker. "Relationship between the Physiochemical Properties of Cocoa Procyanidins and Their Ability to Inhibit Lipid Oxidation in Liposomes." *J Agric Food Chem*, 2018 May: www.ncbi.nlm.nih.gov/pubmed/29649362.

Zeb, A. "Phenolic Profile and Antioxidant Activity of Melon (Cucumis Melo L.) Seeds from Pakistan." *Foods*, 2016 Dec: www.ncbi.nlm.nih.gov/pmc/articles/PMC5302436/.

Photo Credits

Index